MW00441895

MEALS
She
EATS

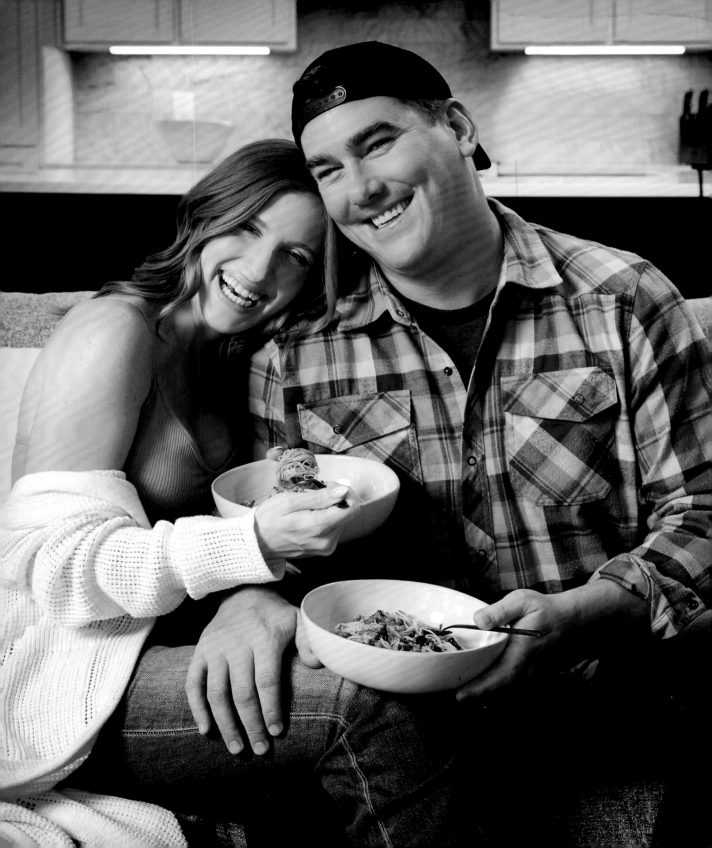

MEALS She EATS

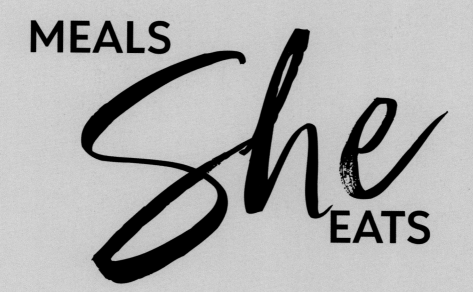

TOM AND RACHAEL SULLIVAN

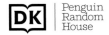 | Penguin Random House

Publisher Mike Sanders
Art & Design Director William Thomas
Senior Editor Alexandra Andrzejewski
Editor Brandon Buechley
Assistant Director of Art/Design Rebecca Batchelor
Technical Editor Bryson Whalen, MD, FACOG
Photographer Kelley Schuyler
Food Stylist for Lifestyle Photography Chung Chow
Food Stylist for Food Photography Lovoni Walker
Recipe Tester Ashley Brooks
Proofreaders Monica Stone, Claire Safran
Indexer Celia McCoy

First American Edition, 2023
Published in the United States by DK Publishing
6081 E. 82nd Street, Suite 400, Indianapolis, IN 46250

Published in the United States by Dorling Kindersley Limited.

Library of Congress Catalog Number: 2022934289
ISBN: 978-0-7440-6493-3

DK books are available at special discounts when purchased in
bulk for sales promotions, premiums, fund-raising, or educational
use. For details, contact: SpecialSales@dk.com.

Printed and bound in China

Photograph on page 192 by Jessi Lancaster Photo

For the curious
www.dk.com

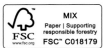

MIX
Paper | Supporting
responsible forestry
FSC™ C018179

This book was made with Forest
Stewardship Council ™ certified
paper – one small step in DK's
commitment to a sustainable future.
**For more information go to
www.dk.com/our-green-pledge**

For those who have PCOS,
who have loved ones with PCOS,
or are significant others to those with PCOS:
this book was created for you.
We are always in your corner and sending our love
to any struggle life throws your way.

For our two biggest fans:
the two people who would be rooting us on
the hardest, the most proud, and standing on
street corners with copies of our book in hand.
We miss you everyday Oonagh Kennedy and
Tom Sullivan.

For our first daughter, Sutton,
you were all the motivation we needed
to take on this journey together . . .
our greatest recipe yet.

CONTENTS

FOREWORD

Journalism is all about telling stories, and for me, those stories have always been my favorite part of the job. I'll never forget scrolling TikTok over my morning coffee and stopping mid scroll to watch a video from Rachael Sullivan. In the video—which has now been viewed over four million times—Rachael shared that she'd found her husband's "secret Instagram account," where he'd been chronicling the PCOS-friendly meals he cooked for her to help regulate her hormones.

Rachael was young, vibrant, beautiful, and full of joy—all in the face of uncertainty surrounding her ability to conceive a child with a man it was clear she loved overwhelmingly. As a mom of two who has cherished making family memories with my own husband, Rachael's candid way of sharing how she was "trying to have little giants" like Tom because there was "nothing she wanted more in life than just to have his babies" struck a chord.

Before my own children were born, I saw friend after friend struggle with infertility and miscarriage. Watching these strong women experience heartbreak each month when the pregnancy test was negative or turn inward to grieve the loss of a pregnancy proved over and over that women are inexplicably strong. When we have the desire to become a mother, we never give up, no matter how that dream takes shape.

I'm a food-and-parenting writer and editor with more than 15 years under my belt, working with outlets like TODAY.com, Reader's Digest, and most recently Yahoo Life. I knew Rachael and Tom's story was special, so I sent them a message before that first morning coffee was finished explaining that I wanted to interview them and do a story on this "secret Instagram." We hopped on the phone, and immediately after the interview, I knew the Sullivans' story would become a part of my life forever.

The first story I wrote about the Sullivans shared their viral TikTok and the @MealsSheEats Instagram account with a new audience. Within days, Tom's "secret account" went from a few followers to a few thousand. I witnessed a phenomenon: people were sharing their own journeys with polycystic ovary syndrome (PCOS) with a couple who immediately made every follower feel like a close friend, if not a member of their family.

And it wasn't just about PCOS. People who menstruate experience many of the same symptoms Rachael was experiencing at some point in their life, from painful hormonal acne to bleeding that's heavy enough to make them call in sick from work and spend the day in bed with their favorite streaming service and a chocolate bar. Periods aren't fun, but the Sullivans were sharing tips and recipes that could possibly make them way more regulated and tolerable, and winning hearts along the way with their beautiful love for one another—and their dog. (Hi, Odin, you good boy.)

In the middle of sharing recipes for lentils in the luteal phase and flaxseed in the follicular phase, the Sullivans found a new passion: cooking these same whole foods–based, cycle–synced meals for North Carolina–area college students. While Rachael, Tom, and I had become forever friends at this point, my journalistic "Spidey sense" tingled again as I watched them share photos of feasts Tom had cooked in their home for young students who were looking for everything from delicious PCOS-friendly dinners to new friends.

And again, because the love of a momma is fierce, the Sullivans started hearing from the *parents* of these college-aged kids who lived thousands of miles away from their children, probably for the first time ever. All a mom wants is for her child to feel accepted, be healthy, and fall asleep each night with a sense of contentment. Using mouthwatering, family-friendly meals like smoked brisket with potato salad or gluten-free spaghetti and meatballs, the Sullivans were taking care of other people's greatest treasures, all while wondering if they'd ever conceive a child of their own.

I interviewed Tom and Rachael again, speaking to them about this newfound passion for helping young adults during one of the most transformative times in their lives. Just like the last time we had a phone conversation, their joy was contagious and their love for one another was a living thing, present on the line.

Amidst their happiness and passion for life (and each other) the Sullivans are also funny—like really funny. Rachael is no pearl-clutcher, sharing stories about everything from considering anal bleaching to navigating online messages from men with foot fetishes. In a world oversaturated with people trying oh so hard to make a name for themselves on social media, it takes a special kind of person to share their life so openly without seeming desperate to elbow their way into the influencer space. Rachael was doing it, and the world was falling in love with the Sullivans's day-to-day lives as much as they were enjoying Tom's recipes.

When Rachael shared her pregnancy news with me, I was overjoyed. Two of the most caring, genuine humans I knew were getting their wish come true, and that was a special thing. I watched Rachael share videos of herself seeing that first positive pregnancy test and telling Tom the news. I cried seeing big, tall Tom turn into a puddle of mushy tears when he heard that Rachael had gotten pregnant, thanks largely to his deep investment in finding out how to use food and recipes to balance his wife's hormones naturally. Again, the Sullivans were giving people hope, one bite at a time.

Few people understand the way food connects to life the way Rachael and Tom do. Because those stunningly beautiful meals Tom had been cooking for years were largely to credit with Rachael's pregnancy, the Sullivans did what they do best—used fresh, colorful whole foods to celebrate the life growing inside of Rachael. Like most of their nearly two million social media followers, I looked forward to weekly posts from the couple where they used food to celebrate the growing baby's size as the pregnancy progressed.

There were pomegranate mocktails when baby Sullivan hit the 17-week mark, carrot noodles at week 21, a rack of ribs at the start of the third trimester, and a naked watermelon photo that nearly broke the internet at week 40. Tom told me he and Rachael both were aware that not all pregnancies result in a living baby, so they decided early on to celebrate every week with their growing little one to make sure they were enjoying their first pregnancy to the fullest, even if the unthinkable happened.

But baby Sullivan grew, and as they did, a deliciously adorable nickname for the baby got cooked up: Torta. Those invested in Rachael and Tom's story embraced the sweet foodie nickname and began sending in "Torta sightings"—photos of everything from tortilla chips to tiny cakes that again connected this couple and their baby to the meals Rachael was eating.

Team "girl" from day one, I wiped away happy tears learning that baby Sutton had arrived safely into the world. This sweet little girl had shown couples struggling with PCOS and infertility that there was hope, and that, *just maybe,* it didn't take a ton of medical intervention to handle those hormones. Again, I watched Tom tearfully look into Rachael's phone camera as he presented "Torta" to the world, answering Rachael's trademark question of *Honey, what do we got?* with news that their long-awaited baby had arrived and she was a little girl.

Sutton's birth meant another interview with the Sullivans. We chatted about the pregnancy, the baby-size weekly foods, and the meaning behind Sutton's name. Of course, there's a food tie. The Sullivans spent their long distance–dating days meeting halfway at a Kentucky restaurant called Sutton's, named for the owner's daughter. They shared that the name had stuck, even then. Through dating, married life, a PCOS diagnosis, and trying to conceive, baby Sutton's name was tucked inside their hearts—more evidence that this beautiful couple was destined to be amazing parents from the beginning.

As someone who has watched the Sullivans' incredible story unfold from early on, seeing the *Meals She Eats* book come to fruition feels like the obvious next step and almost as much a cause for celebration as the birth of their daughter. After all, they wrote this book *and* grew a baby simultaneously.

Those followers the couple has gained along the way can now follow along with the family's food journey in a different way—keeping a complete guide to PCOS, a cycle-syncing diet, and Tom's most trusted recipes in the kitchen with them, no cell phone required.

In *Meals She Eats,* the Sullivans share parts of their story you may have missed, along with Rachael's own personal experience with PCOS, irregular periods, and hormone regulation through food. This cookbook-meets-PCOS-handbook will teach you how to eat in sync with your menstrual cycle and reap all the delicious benefits of doing so.

That's not all you'll find in the pages of this book. Through the information, personal anecdotes, and delicious recipes the Sullivans share, you'll find hope. Whether you're facing a PCOS diagnosis, feeling the devastation of infertility, or wondering if true love exists, *Meals She Eats* will give you the tools (and mood boost) you need to take charge of your health and jump head first into working on making your dreams a reality, all while enjoying stunning colorful photos of some of Rachael's favorite recipes and saying *aww* at seriously sweet shots of the couple in their kitchen.

Meals She Eats ushers in a brave new world where people who menstruate do not have to be passive participants in getting their period. Rachael's candor in sharing her initial PCOS symptoms and how she reversed them through Tom's specialized way of cooking is proof that we no longer need to submit to irregular hormones, unnaturally heavy bleeding, and a face full of painful period-related acne.

Do other books on the topic of food and hormones exist? Yes. But none are as intermixed with love, family, and joy as this guide, developed by some of the most genuinely kind humans I've ever known. Turning the pages of *Meals She Eats* will make you feel like you're dining (and learning) with Rachael and Tom, just like one of the college students the Sullivans routinely welcome into their home.

So pull up a chair in the Sullivans' kitchen and enjoy some pork stew. Tom's had it on the stove for hours.

–Terri Peters
Senior Lifestyle Editor, *Yahoo Life*

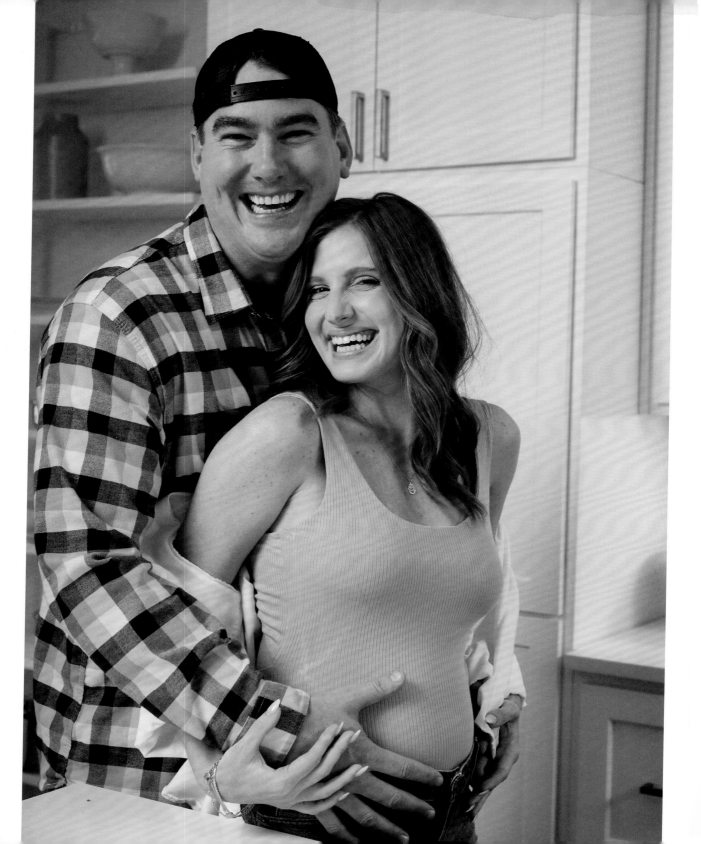

INTRODUCTION

The day we found out we were pregnant was the same day we got a book deal. It was surreal. At that point, Rachael's menstrual cycle, which was once lost, had been restored—now a 32-day cycle, ovulating in rhythm, for 14 months straight. Other symptoms that used to weigh on us both for years seemed like a distant thought. But there was still a big question mark in our lives: could we get pregnant? Before that magical stick turned blue, we worried whether we'd have difficulty conceiving, even after all that hard work regulating her cycle. We were talking about making fertility appointments for the both of us, just to be proactive. We were debating if all this PCOS therapy was worth it if we couldn't reach our end goal. (Which was silly because the lifestyle truly changed both of our lives for the better, pregnancy or not.) Getting the news that the book deal was on while sobbing over the thought of becoming parents was truly a moment that will live with us forever.

We have thought long and hard about what *you* want from this book. We are neither doctors nor nutritionists, but we have been researching and implementing our research for years with amazing results. During that time, we have formed relationships with numerous doctors, some who take a holistic approach, as well as others who take a conventional approach to managing PCOS. We have worked closely with the National Polycystic Ovary Syndrome Association as well as a multitude of experts in the PCOS field. It has been amazing to see the growth of our PCOS community on social media and a truly humbling feeling to receive testimonials from so many people who menstruate as they use our methods to reach their goals. We are thrilled to share our research and experiences with you.

This book is a mixture of our personalities. Rachael is fun, whimsical, honest (nearly to a fault,) and passionate. Tom loves to cook, and it's important to him to understand the how and why for just about everything he encounters. We share details about our lives that led us here, insights we have learned about PCOS, some of the heartaches and ways to avoid them, foods we enjoy, and tips and tricks in between. There are some heavy medical pieces in our book that Tom obsesses over, right down to discussing menstrual blood color and cervical mucus. And of course we hope the recipes become family staples. We tried to pick out dishes that are significant to our lives and do the double duty of helping heal the body. Many of these recipes have even been incorporated into our meals-to-go gatherings we started in 2021 after "adopting" thousands of college students by inviting them into our home for home-cooked meals.

While this is a book about PCOS, anyone who wants to get healthier can certainly take away lots. Tom doesn't menstruate, but he has seen huge improvements in his quality of life by following this lifestyle. We hope that you are able to understand a bit about what happens in the body when you have PCOS, therapies to combat it, and some very realistic ways to start. Honestly, Rachael's iconic stories alone (her first period or tampon experience!) make this book worth reading.

–TOM AND RACH

HOW IT ALL STARTED

RACHAEL: I've always trusted Tom to not keep any secrets from me. That was until the day I found out about his second Instagram account. It's not that I really found the account either . . . the account found me. There's a section on Instagram called "People You May Know," and there was my husband's name and profile picture with the account name *MealsSheEats*. Any sane woman who just found her husband's hidden social media account might internally scream, *"Who the hell is this SHE?"* and I did just that. I opened the account, but instead of finding a secret life with a secret wife, I found several photos of the previous week's dinner. The first photo was miso soup with the caption "Great for hormonal balance during that time of the month, aka keep her happy.... #pcos #pcosfood #misosoup #guthealing #holisticnutrition"

The entire page was dedicated to recipes to help balance my hormones! When I was diagnosed with PCOS the previous year and we realized this could impact our chances to start a family, we changed the way we approach food. So yes, when I saw those little hashtags, my heart was bursting.

TOM: In fairness, it was a secret so I could save Rachael from herself; our food would get cold because she would inevitably produce a photo shoot to feature the food on the Insta page. In practice, I just needed a place to put a picture, my recipe, and some thoughts. The former system of not measuring ingredients, having loose thoughts in my notes app, disorganized Pinterest boards, browser bookmarks, and random saved Instagram posts wasn't going to cut it. I wanted to be able to officially chronicle every ingredient I

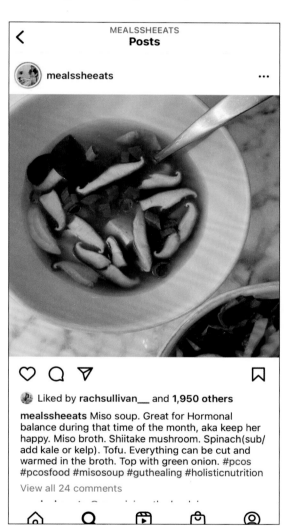

used in a dish, as well as look back at meals she liked during certain phases of her cycle. Instagram seemed like the easiest and quickest place to document all this. What's funny is I didn't tell her about the Instagram account out of fear of her always wanting to take pretty pictures, when in fact the moment she stops to take a photo of a plate I just put in front of her, it is the best feeling in the world. It's the Rachael stamp of approval.

RACHAEL: A week later, I made a TikTok video about the Instagram discovery, and Tom's sweet gesture went viral overnight, reaching four million views. His Instagram account grew from 79 followers to over 5,000 followers in a matter of hours. *That was a lot of random people who now knew exactly when I was menstruating.* Later that week, we got a DM from a woman named Terri with the *TODAY Show* asking if we'd be up for an interview. It would be for the TODAY.com food section.

"They want to write a story about us?" Tom asked.

Did we just read that right? We took the phone interview in a parking lot just outside Asheville, North Carolina, before heading into the mountains for what was supposed to be a quiet, unplugged evening with no cell service. That night turned into anything but—the *TODAY Show* featured our interview not only in the food section, but also as a headline story. We were plastered on the homepage, and it began to circulate around several other news pages. I'll never forget that our article

was inches away from Matt Damon's face on Flipboard. That same week, we got a voicemail from a number we didn't recognize: "Hey Tom, my name is Erin. I work for the *Rachael Ray Show*. Um, I came across a story about you and your wife and wanted to chat with you to learn a little bit more." I remember we both looked at each other thinking *What the hell is happening?*

TOM: Did I think this was going to happen? Not a chance. In a 48-hour window, the following of @mealssheeats went from double digits to thousands. Suddenly, I had all these people watching *me* . . . was I expected to, like, make content? I don't even think I'd ever posted an Instagram Story up until that point.

RACHAEL: As Tom's account grew, there were also more and more people coming to the page who were in the same situation as me: women who had PCOS, might have PCOS, women who were unsure but knew something was off with their bodies, and women trying to start a family but it wasn't happening. As Tom began receiving more and more messages, we began learning how big of an issue managing PCOS really was. Then the messages flooded in about people feeling hopeful and realizing they weren't alone, and the gratitude they expressed was overwhelming.

Saying that PCOS is underresourced is an understatement. We started to dedicate more time to recipes, research, and resources. It was becoming a full-time job, and Tom's employers had been giving him a hard time ever since the airing of Rachael Ray, often questioning where his time was going. It came to the point where we hit a fork in the road that required some deep conversations. *How can we keep both up? Can we turn away from something that has become a passion? Isn't this what people dream of finding? But can you even "do" social media full time?*

A few months later, we posted an "Ask Us Anything" question box on social media, and someone asked if we were ever going to write a cookbook. I told Tom to repost it and say, "Sure! Does anyone know a publisher?" because I'm a big believer in manifesting and putting your desires out to the universe.

Days later, we were approached about this very lifestyle book, and it was a full-circle moment from where we started to how far we'd come. We took it as a sign for Tom to leave his current career path in medical sales to really focus on something more fulfilling. This book has allowed us to look back on our journey that started way before social media and even dating. It's a journey of love, passion, hardship, and understanding, and we're so grateful to be able to share this with you.

GETTING IN TUNE WITH MY BODY

I lived in a household where we weren't allowed to drink caffeinated Pepsi or Coke, but a can of Orange Crush or Sprite was okay. A bagel with cream cheese wasn't considered a healthy breakfast option, but for some reason a bowl of Fruity Pebbles was. There was a disconnect between food choices and how they affect the body. (In defense of my mother, I will say that her antics to keep us at arm's length from caffeine worked. I never was one to rely on a cup of coffee or an energy drink to get me through the day.) However, our joint ignorance about the effects that sugar played in the body had a crippling effect on my future.

By my senior year of high school, I had stopped being an active athlete burning 1500 calories a day at soccer practice. Instead, I was an inactive high schooler holding onto my old eating habits that used to sustain my energy throughout the day—but now without the consistency of an active sports schedule. I subsisted on cheese-stuffed breadsticks and pizza puffs, followed by a bag of Jolly Ranchers for lunch. I started to gain weight and feel extremely unhealthy in my body. I wanted to take better care of myself, but mentally, I couldn't find the motivation to do so.

After deciding not to try out for the varsity soccer team for fear of not making the cut, I lost my drive and determination to push myself. Reading over that line makes me sad. *I was so afraid of not making the cut that I didn't even give myself a chance.* This will be an important lesson as you move forward with your journey to managing your PCOS: you aren't doing yourself any favors by being afraid to try something new that may seem a little scary to you. I began cutting corners as a way to make life simpler.

Instead of incorporating exercise into my daily routine, I was introduced to the easy way out: calorie counting or the principle of burning more calories than you eat in order to lose weight. Why focus on the foods that offered the nutrients my body needed when I could eat 1,700 calories of whatever I wanted and still lose or manage my weight? I didn't understand the concept of "food is fuel." For lunch, I began swapping out my pizza puffs for a salad; that way I could still eat a bag of candy and be under my daily threshold of calories. I didn't understand that the huge daily amount of sugar I was consuming was poison for my body. The initial swap from pizza to salads was an excellent start, but salads don't necessarily equate to being the "healthiest" option, as you will learn. Despite all of this, I was working toward a health goal, and that was a start.

By the time I got to college, counting calories was exhausting, and I needed a new approach to food. College is the time for exploration, as they say, and for me this meant becoming a vegetarian. This wasn't some religious conviction or because of some politically moving documentary I watched. Nor did it have to do with my desire to save the planet. I was just 19 years old and wanted to figure out what diet worked best with my body. My roommate was also a vegetarian, so she made the transition less daunting by helping me with meal prep. She was my Yoda and I was her Luke Skywalker. (The fact that I actually just referenced *Star Wars* is comical because I am not a fan, but Tom is and I know that'll put a smile on his face.) I had one overarching goal here and that was the desire to learn to love vegetables. This transition also took place around the time I started dating Tom.

TOM ENTERS THE CHAT

There are a lot of moments in our relationship that reinforced the belief that Tom was the man for me. For example take our first conversation via DM. He asked what I was studying in college, and I said I was going to take a different route in life. I flirted that I would marry rich, experience all the finer things I could never afford myself, and write a memoir about it. Sounded like a solid plan, right? Tom then joked he had a similar plan but it didn't work out in his favor, so now he was going to be the one to make "dat" bread. Without hesitation, I offered my hand in marriage and said if he got rich, I'd be honored to call him my husband one day. I then tried to seal the deal with the irresistible notion that I could make a mad bowl of cereal anytime, on demand: "It's all about that perfect milk ratio that some people can't seem to master." I then guaranteed there would never be a dull moment in his life. He agreed that he struggled with the cereal thing, which until this moment I didn't question to be true—but now that I think about it, Tom still struggles with the proper ratio for making rice, so maybe he was telling the truth. He said, "I'm not going to lie. I am one hell of a good cook so I can take care of that end of the deal."

Sometimes the first DM or conversation can be all talk, but Tom held to his end of the deal. I spent a week of my summer with him that year in southern Illinois, and the man cooked all vegetarian for me. Little did I know Tom had never made a main dish without animal

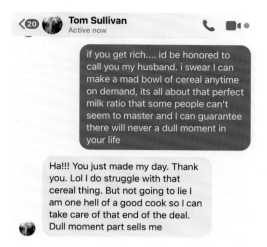

protein before, but he was smitten by me, so he wasn't going to admit that.

My vegetarian lifestyle only lasted a few months—I really couldn't go without barbecue or bacon—but since day one, Tom's been conscious of my dietary needs and always has the utmost respect when it comes to honoring how I choose to nurture my body.

It comes as no surprise that when I wanted to try out Whole30 before our wedding, Tom didn't skip a beat. He even joined me. Whole30 is an elimination diet created by Dallas Hartwig and Melissa Urban. The program asks you to look at *everything* you put into your mouth. For 30 days, we completely avoided inflammatory foods that were known to trigger immune responses within the body. This included all forms of added sugar, grains, dairy, gluten, and alcohol as a way to "reset" the body. (Don't tell Melissa, but we did still enjoy wine with meals here and there.) After 2 weeks, I already could feel a change in my body, and after a month, I was a whole new me. All of the awful symptoms that had crept in since high school were changing. My sleep patterns were better, and I had more energy. I started to notice major improvements in my acne. Up until that point, I always dealt with horrible bloating and thought it was just what everyone felt after they ate. When we started to reintroduce foods into my body, I felt uncomfortable in my own skin, and those painful stomach cramps came creeping back in. I specifically remember drinking a Blue Moon beer and immediately feeling pain in my stomach. It became very apparent there was something I was consuming that caused these uncomfortable symptoms—I just wasn't completely sure what that was.

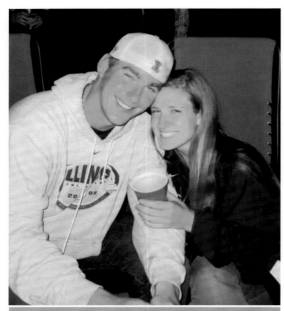

EARLY DATING! THIS WAS MY FIRST NFL TAILGATE.

MY PCOS JOURNEY

It wasn't until 2019 that I made a doctor's appointment leading to the shocking discovery that my hormones were linked to the food I was eating. Since we got married, we weren't necessarily trying for a baby, but we were also not *not* trying. I also had a history of irregular periods, but it never bothered me until the thought of starting a family. I was more than happy skipping a month or two of being trapped in bed with debilitating cramps and a heating pad and the embarrassing notion of having to sleep on a towel so I didn't bleed onto the sheets. I had an inkling I might have PCOS because of a girl on social media who shared her journey. She had irregular and painful periods, facial hair, and acne. If this was PCOS I was dealing with, I wanted to get ahead of it because one of the side effects included trouble conceiving.

When I mentioned I thought it was PCOS, my doctor was very dismissive. She said she had PCOS, which was "no big deal." The way she minimized my concerns made them feel invalid. She also recommended I go on hormonal birth control to regulate my cycle, which is a whole different facet to the story. Nevertheless, I had blood work done that day and a vaginal ultrasound later that week. They concluded that I did have cystic ovaries and hormone imbalances, confirming a diagnosis of PCOS. I cried in the bathroom of our rental unit when I got the news, not because I was upset, but because for the first time I didn't feel totally crazy. There was an underlying health condition that I was dealing with, and now the only thing left to figure out was how to tackle it.

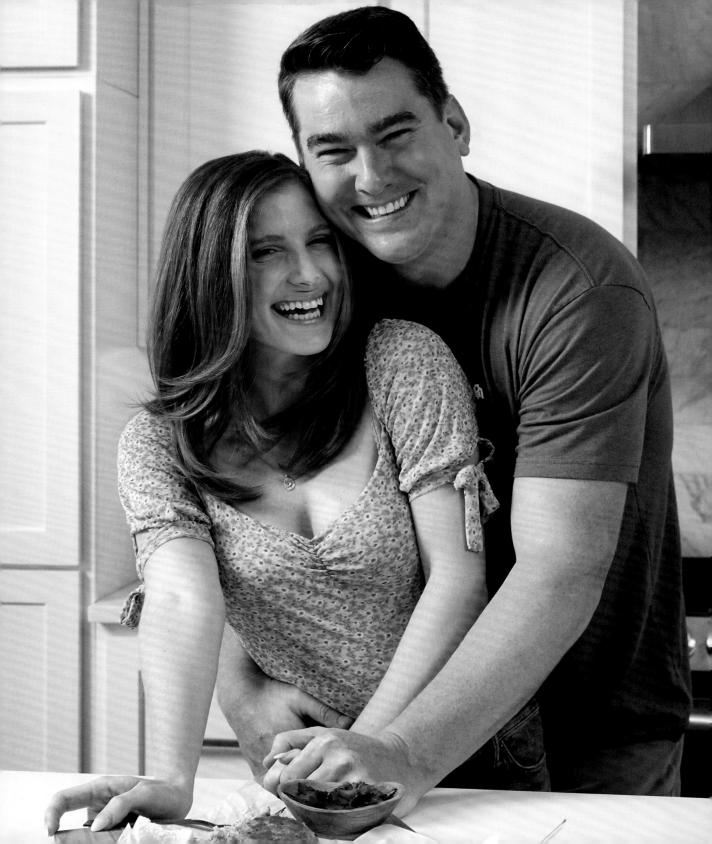

PART 1

UNDERSTAND AND NAVIGATE

When people speak of medical care, several things may come to mind—most generally doctors and hospitals. By far the most common question we receive is, "How do I find the right doctor?" It's typically followed by a story of being dismissed by one along their journey. When managing PCOS, it's important to realize that care goes beyond just the traditional medical field. It also needs to include nutritional help, physical activity, and mental health. This isn't to overwhelm you, but rather to acknowledge that medical, nutritional, physical, and mental health in many ways have been separated into their own categories, when in a perfect world these fields would overlap on a regular basis and work together.

The medical side of things is vital for understanding what is going on with your body, deciding what labs you may need to run, monitoring progress, and considering medication when it's needed. Physical activity helps with weight control, happiness, and overall quality of life. The nutritional-health side provides the nutrient stability our bodies need to stay fueled, energized, and healthy. Lastly, mental health overlaps with all of these. We are dealing with hormone imbalances, after all. Imbalances change our mental states, physical states, and emotional states, day by day. It was important for both of us that this book bring light to each of these fields while adding our own personal experiences.

When laying out this book, it was essential for us to have a set of eyes on the medical side. We wanted guidance from someone who provides informed and thoughtful care for PCOS patients daily and who could speak plainly with us about the medical aspects of this complex syndrome. Bryson Whalen MD, FACOG, was a clear fit as a medical expert who is passionate about the topic.

I was so excited when Tom and Rachael reached out to me to be a part of this project. I saw this book as a great tool in an area of my practice that had a great void. A lot of medical literature lists lifestyle modifications, including diet and exercise, as the cornerstones of treatment for PCOS. However, the majority of medical providers have a very peripheral knowledge of exercise, physiology, and nutrition. We may recommend these things to our patients, but we may not be the best at coaching in these arenas. Because of this, it's often perceived by patients that "my doctor just gave me pills and didn't explain anything." I hope this book reminds providers about the importance of counseling and educating our patients on the challenging diagnosis they are facing. Informing and educating the patient is an important part of practicing medicine and may take several visits to fully cover all the different aspects of the diagnosis. This book should encourage providers to be open to the idea of adapting a team approach to treating PCOS and reaching out to other health professionals, such as nutritionists and psychologists. As medical providers, it's easy to get into routines or develop habits when we deal with specific problems over and over again. Let's keep in mind that PCOS is a complex diagnosis, and each patient's experience with PCOS will be unique. I hope any medical providers who read this book will use it as a tool for open discussion with patients regarding every aspect of PCOS and will allow them to think outside of the box when considering treatment options. I also hope women with PCOS who read this book feel empowered to take control of their lifestyle to improve their well-being while dealing with the challenges of this syndrome. –Dr. Bryson Whalen

CHAPTER 1

AN OVERVIEW OF PCOS

TOM: Polycystic ovary syndrome (PCOS) is a complicated condition, and it's something that a women's health care provider is likely to encounter daily. Not monthly—daily. Conservative estimates show that about 8 percent of women have PCOS, whether they've been diagnosed or not, and more liberal estimates say that 18 percent of women have the condition.* So when you feel like you are going through this battle alone, you aren't. Countless other women are in your shoes right now, reading this book for the same exact reasons. They, too, want to manage this choke hold that PCOS has over every aspect of their lives, their bodies, their relationships, their minds, their sex drives, and their overall quality of life. First, it's important to understand what exactly PCOS is from a medical standpoint.

WHAT IS PCOS?

PCOS is a dysfunction of the female reproductive system resulting in increased male hormones, irregular menstrual cycles, and insulin resistance. Remember a few seconds ago when I told you that you aren't alone? PCOS is the most common endocrine disorder in women and one of the leading causes of infertility. Despite how common it is, it remains a challenge for providers and patients to diagnose and understand.

> ## PCOS is the most common endocrine disorder in women and one of the leading causes of infertility.

DEFINING

Defining PCOS is an important part of understanding both the diagnosis and the treatment. As the name implies, PCOS is a syndrome, not a disease. A *syndrome* is a collection of symptoms associated with a specific health condition without an identifiable cause; whereas a *disease* is the body's response to specific, known internal or external factors. Because PCOS is a collection of varying symptoms, there is no universal definition for PCOS. Crazy, right? Millions of women suffer from PCOS, but it's clear much more research needs to be dedicated to it.

---

* March, W. A., V. M. Moore, K. J. Willson, D. I.W. Phillips, R. J. Norman, and M. J. Davies. "The Prevalence of Polycystic Ovary Syndrome in a Community Sample Assessed under Contrasting Diagnostic Criteria." *Human Reproduction* 25, no. 2 (November 12, 2009): 544–51. https://doi.org/10.1093/humrep/dep399.

Providers use certain criteria to establish the diagnosis (see *Diagnosing PCOS* on page 35). There are several professional societies that have published their own criteria, and each varies in their definitions. These criteria are very loose and include a broad list of common symptoms for women, and that's where things get complicated. This lack of clarity in definition and varying diagnostic criteria can lead to over- and underdiagnosing the syndrome amongst varying providers. Consider the fact that not all women with PCOS have ovarian cysts and not all women with ovarian cysts have PCOS. I mean, the name of the syndrome is *polycystic ovary syndrome,* so to realize that you don't even need to have ovarian cysts to be diagnosed with PCOS illustrates just how complex this diagnosis can be.

RISKS AND SYMPTOMS

These are main symptoms/signs you can physically see or feel that are red flags for PCOS:

1. Painful or heavy periods

2. Irregular periods

3. No period

4. Weight gain

5. Hormonal acne

6. Sleep irregularities or constant fatigue

Rachael's Christmas Miracle

A Christmas miracle *was all I thought as I sat on the toilet on December 25 and realized the moment of becoming a woman was happening. For years, when alone in the bathroom, I would stuff my shirt with toilet paper in anticipation of seeing what having boobs would look like on me. My mother didn't get her period until she was a freshman in high school, so while my friends in sixth grade were experiencing this whole new chapter in their lives, I knew it might take me a few years to catch up. Getting my period was something I had been looking forward to as long as I could remember. There was no lack of preparation for this moment. By eighth grade, I was still holding onto that blue sparkly purse—filled with tampons and mini pads, given to me in a sex education class years prior—that was collecting dust at the bottom of my closet. I also spent that entire last summer wearing a mini pad every day to harness the rituals of womanhood . . . and because I was known to leak if I laughed too hard.*

7. Excess body hair growth

8. Male-pattern hair loss

9. Infertility

10. Decreased sex drive

While these are the main symptoms, it is fairly common to not show all of these symptoms and still have PCOS. Unexplained physical changes might be PCOS, but they could also be something else, and at the end of the day your health is most important. You know your body best and if you feel like something is off, talk to your doctor.

THE HEALTHY MENSTRUAL CYCLE

To better understand PCOS, let's first establish an understanding of the "healthy" menstrual cycle. This was not something kids were taught in grade school, so get ready for your 200–level course analysis on all things menstruation.

The brain and the ovaries control the menstrual cycle: the cycle of releasing an egg and building up the uterine lining, which then sheds during bleeding or your period. When the brain sends hormonal signals to the ovaries, the ovaries respond to the signals by producing two important hormones: estrogen and progesterone. These two hormones directly affect the lining of the uterus.

Throughout the book, we will refer to the menstrual cycle in four phases: menstrual, follicular, ovulatory, and luteal. It's important to note from a medical perspective that the menstrual cycle is in fact only broken down into two phases: the follicular and luteal phases with the *events* of ovulation and menstruation falling into each phase. Don't let that make your head spin. In order to help you better understand the hormonal fluctuations and how they are responsible for transitioning the body from one phase to the next, we will be referring to each event as its own specific phase. These phases are characterized by the effects of the hormonal signals from the ovaries. (More on those hormones in a bit.) In a healthy cycle, you'll see the four phases shown in the diagram to the right.

THE FOUR PHASES

A typical, healthy cycle follows these four phases. In reality, the length of each phase or event varies from person to person.

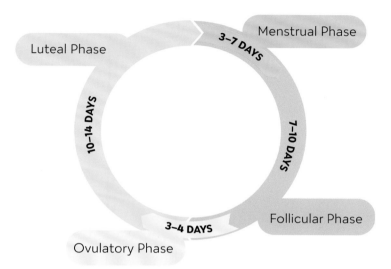

Luteal Phase

Menstrual Phase

3–7 DAYS

10–14 DAYS

7–10 DAYS

Follicular Phase

3–4 DAYS

Ovulatory Phase

MENSTRUAL PHASE

This is when bleeding begins. The uterus sheds its lining (called menses) so that the cycle can begin.

OVULATORY PHASE

This event is the release of the egg from the dominant follicle. The released egg gets picked up into the fallopian tube and subsequently passes through the uterus. This usually occurs midmenstrual cycle and signifies the start of the luteal phase. The follicle that held the released egg becomes the corpus luteum, a temporary hormone-producing gland that sticks around in your ovary throughout the luteal phase to produce progesterone. It disintegrates by the next period.

FOLLICULAR PHASE

It begins as your period ends. The ovaries gradually grow a few eggs into a large follicle in preparation for the event called ovulation. Typically one or two follicles will grow the largest and become the "dominant follicles." The uterine lining also begins to thicken during this phase in preparation for possible implantation of an embryo in the lining.

LUTEAL PHASE

This phase begins immediately after the egg is released. As the egg travels through the uterus, the uterine lining continues to thicken into a nutritive place for a fertilized egg to implant if pregnancy occurs. If pregnancy doesn't occur, hormones drop and the next period begins.

KEY CYCLE HORMONES

The hypothalamic-pituitary-ovarian (HPO) axis is an endocrine system through which several hormones communicate with each other to produce your menstrual cycle. When we experience symptoms of hormonal imbalance it can be because one or many of these hormones have gone out of balance, leading to PCOS.

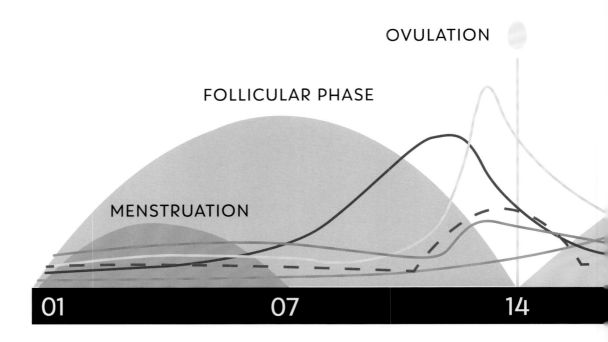

Estrogen, *produced primarily in the ovaries, develops and maintains the body, including breasts, strong bones, healthy heart, and even sex drive. It also helps build the uterine lining in preparation for potential pregnancy. The primary type of estrogen is called* estradiol, *and it surges and peaks during the follicular phase, although it should stick around in moderate amounts during the luteal phase, as well.*

Progesterone, *produced by the corpus luteum in the ovaries, is a leading hormone that prepares your body for and sustains pregnancy. It produces a number of general, positive health effects. Proper amounts of progesterone have calming effects on your body, working to reduce premenstrual syndrome and anxiety. It's like a natural antidepressant. Your body can only produce adequate progesterone when you've ovulated. Its presence counteracts estrogen for balanced hormones.*

LUTEAL PHASE

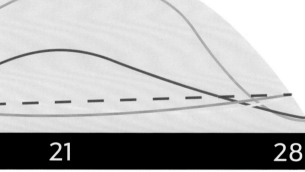

21   28

Follicle-stimulating hormone (FSH) *stimulates the follicle to begin maturing and elevates estrogen production. Its sharp rise contributes to a mature follicle and ovulation. It's produced in the pituitary gland, which is part of the brain's hypothalamic region.*

Luteinizing hormone (LH) *typically elevates right before ovulation, causing the egg to release and ovulation to begin. LH also helps with the production of progesterone, making it essential for maintaining a regular cycle. LH is also produced in the pituitary gland.*

Testosterone and DHEA-S, *produced in the ovaries and adrenal glands, are androgens (male hormones) that are necessary in relatively low levels to help regulate the cycle. Excess levels can produce male-characteristic symptoms (acne, hair loss, and hirsutism), as well as classic PCOS symptoms.*

THE PCOS MENSTRUAL CYCLE

In women with PCOS, the hormonal system does not work in perfect orchestration because of three main factors: (1) increased LH, (2) increased androgens, and (3) insulin resistance. These are consistent, key findings, leading to a vicious cycle of ripple effects.

1. The excess secretion of LH—the brain's signal to the ovaries to trigger ovulation—overwhelms the hormone production of the ovaries and, in effect, leads to increased circulation of androgens.

Let's zoom in to get a more detailed picture. Imagine hormone production in the ovaries like a factory with an assembly line. Usually the body would take those androgens and convert them to estrogen, but the assembly line cannot keep up with the demands to convert this excess androgen. In effect, inappropriate levels of the male hormones leak through the system, leading to the rise in circulating androgens that cause your PCOS.

2. Excess androgens impair the ability for a single, dominant follicle to mature for ovulation. In turn, many follicles (*far* too many for some women) are stimulated to grow, but all are frozen in mid-development without any emerging as candidates for ovulation. These many follicles give the ovaries their polycystic (many cysts) appearance.

Without a dominant follicle, when the brain signals to ovulate, no egg is released. This also

THE VICIOUS CYCLE OF PCOS

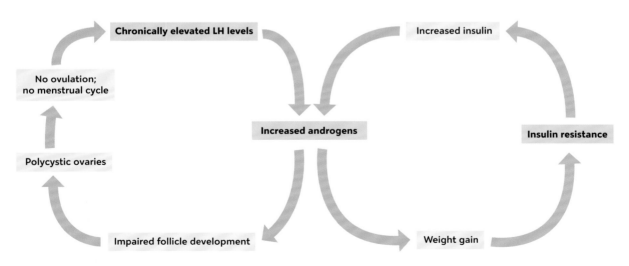

means that progesterone is not produced in the luteal phase. Without the rise and subsequent fall of progesterone, there is no shedding of the uterine lining during menses.

3. Insulin is a metabolic hormone released by the pancreas to help the body use the carbs you eat, thereby keeping your blood sugar at a healthy level. Since the body is resistant to its own insulin in PCOS, the body produces *more* insulin to achieve its effects. The exact cause of the resistance isn't clear, but it could be a combination of weight gain, poorly controlled blood sugar (frequent highs and lows), low physical activity levels, and genetics. This excess insulin acts on the brain to increase its signals to the ovaries, which further increases the development of androgens and immature follicles.

You can see how this vicious cycle repeats and has a compounding effect on itself.

Maybe most of this section went right over your head—don't worry about it! I love to know why things work and what is happening. Rachael loves to dive into remedies and learn through trial and error. The combination of both is how we found what works best for our lifestyle together.

DIAGNOSING PCOS

Not all doctors agree with which combination of criteria warrants a PCOS diagnosis, but the most commonly used criteria is called the *Rotterdam criteria,* which requires the presence of at least two of three conditions: hyperandrogenism (excess androgens), oligomenorrhea (irregular or infrequent periods), and polycystic ovaries (a high cyst count on the ovaries).

ROTTERDAM CRITERIA

Two of these three criteria warrant a diagnosis of PCOS.

Elevated androgens	Typically shown by high testosterone or DHEA-S levels in the blood, or through physical signs of hormonal imbalance, such as increased hair growth on the face or body.
Irregular periods	Less than 21 days or more than 35 days between periods.
High cyst count on the ovaries	Typically 12 or more follicles—each measuring 2 to 9mm in diameter—on one ovary. In other words, the quantity and size matter. You might hear this called "the string of pearls." Having cysts on your ovaries is not a sure sign of PCOS, but by the same token, you could be cyst-free and still be diagnosed with PCOS.

DIAGNOSTIC FAQS

Q: Is an ultrasound necessary?

A: Not all the time. A vaginal ultrasound will allow your doctor to scan the follicles in your ovaries to see if they're polycystic. However, you could display enough strong signs of PCOS without needing to check the ovaries; then you can simply begin your treatment journey. That being said, your doctor may still order one, and you can always request one.

Q: What labs should I get done?

A: Medical professionals look at labs as a way to set some baselines for monitoring PCOS and your overall health. They also identify areas where you potentially need help.

Some recommended labs are...

- *Reproductive hormones:* FSH, LH, estradiol, progesterone, anti-Mullerian hormone (AMH).

- *Androgens:* total and free testosterone, DHEA-S.

- *Metabolic:* hemoglobin A1C, fasting insulin, cholesterol panel, comprehensive metabolic panel, oral glucose tolerance test (OGTT).

- *Other:* full thyroid panel, vitamin D.

Q: What if my doctor does not think labs are necessary?

A: Well, they may *not* be necessary or necessary *at this time,* but you should have a doctor you trust and who is right for you and open to the discussion. Some people like a doctor telling them what is needed; some like overexplaining. We are all different in terms of our personalities. If you print this list and walk into the doctor's office stating "Tom and Rachael said you should be running these tests" . . . well, first the doctor will wonder who the heck Tom and Rachael are and then probably be turned off to having you as a patient. It does go both ways. Now, if you state that you have read about these tests and wondered if they might benefit you, the way the doctor answers this will probably give you a feel if they are the right doctor for you.

Why "Fix" Your PCOS?

Maybe you're experiencing absent or "skipped" periods and view it as a luxury! So why should you work on correcting the many symptoms of your PCOS? Due to the hormonal imbalance and dysfunction seen in PCOS, there is an increased risk for several long-term health consequences. Women with PCOS are at increased risk of issues such as infertility, endometrial cancer, obesity, elevated blood pressure, obesity-related cardiovascular disease, sleep apnea, diabetes, and depression. Plus, you're probably realizing some of the more overt and debilitating symptoms of PCOS noted in this chapter. Changing some of your lifestyle factors could really help mitigate those symptoms.

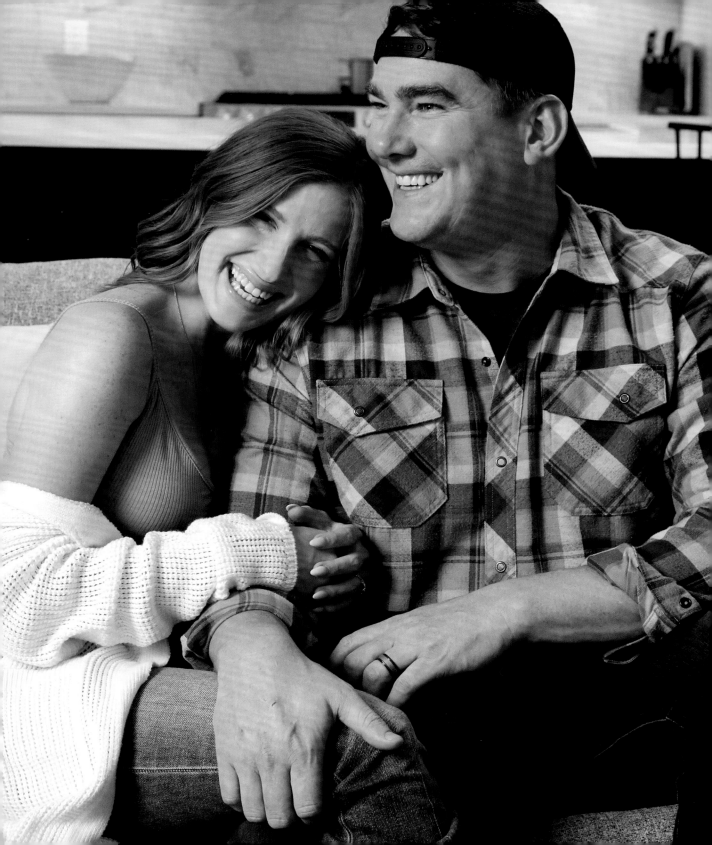

CHAPTER 2

SO YOU HAVE PCOS

RACHAEL: We hope your mind isn't drowning in menstrual knowledge and diagnosis particulars. Let's say you *do* have PCOS, whether by official diagnosis or not—take a deep breath. We will help you navigate some of your next steps, such as starting a journal and finding the right doctor who supports your goals. We are building a lifestyle around feeling great despite our diagnosis, so let's explore some practical ways to start your PCOS journey.

JOURNALING YOUR SYMPTOMS AND SIGNS

It is unbelievably helpful to write in a journal or take notes in an app on your phone daily. Start to track what is happening with your body. This will keep you objective and take the guesswork out of your signs and symptoms as days, weeks, or even months go by.

To this day, the expectation of the patterns brings me peace because I feel more attuned with my body and less surprised by symptoms and signs.

As you've discovered, having PCOS means your hormones aren't perfectly orchestrated. Like the melody to your favorite song, you need each instrument to play a different part, ideally in sync, to sound harmonized. When even the slightest note is off key, you can expect the song to sound a little off. This is the same for your body. Maybe there's a

Getting It On Record

Before journaling, I was a basket case when it came to understanding my emotions and my body. Part of me would block out those repeated feelings of anxiety, irritability, and depression because, let's be honest—no one wants to dwell on negative feelings after they've passed. And every cycle, Tom would gently point out the recurring patterns so that I could be less surprised by them. Maybe it's because he was observing from the outside looking in, but he was more prepared for the shift my body would undergo than I was. Once I stopped internalizing all my emotions and started documenting them, I was able to save myself from the emotional turmoil I was putting myself through.

sudden flare up in your acne or a "missed" menstrual cycle. Whatever the problem may be, this is your body indicating that perhaps there's something out of tune that needs evaluating. This knowledge is powerful information you can provide your doctor with to discuss or tweak some lifestyle habits to get you back on beat.

Journal what your long-term and short-term goals are for your health. Don't be afraid to share them with your doctor either. For example, when we had a goal to start a family, you can see why being offered to take the pill to alleviate my PMS symptoms didn't align with that goal. Goals can range anywhere from starting a family to seeing improvements in your lab work that directly correlate to your health and a lessening of unwanted symptoms (such as increased progesterone or lowered HbA1c), or to staying hydrated throughout the day. These are your goals, so make them as broad or specific as you want. My first health goal was to walk 100 miles, a number that seemed daunting. Yet with actionable steps (see what I did there) it seemed less and less out of reach. If I could walk an average of 3 miles a day, 100 miles was no longer an impossible task and one that could be accomplished within several weeks.

There are countless apps and even paper charts out there to keep track of everything. I use an app called Flo to track my sex drive, how often we have sex, mood, vaginal discharge/cervical mucus, and several other symptoms and signs. A few other great app options include Read Your Body, Kindara, and Clue. Find one that fits your needs.

Specific methods of cycle tracking and interpretation are a complex topic and deserve a whole book (and there are some great ones out there for this purpose). We will not dive into the particulars of how to interpret your cycle using fertility-awareness methods, but what we offer will help you to keep general awareness and give you some ideas to discuss with your doctor. If fertility-awareness methods interest you, there is a whole world of content (books, groups, podcasts, programs, etc.) that you can learn from, and you can even work with instructors or doctors who specialize in a method.

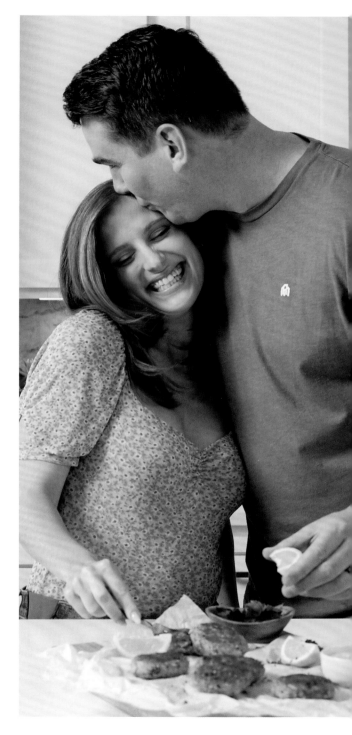

SIGNS AND SYMPTOMS TO RECORD

Here are some of the signs and symptoms we recommend recording on a daily basis. A sample journal is found on the next page.

CYCLE (MENSTRUATION)

Monitor every day of your cycle, noting whether you're spotting, on your period, or have a vaginal discharge of some sort. Record the qualities of any cervical fluid you observe, as well as your menstrual blood's color and weight or volume. These signs point to important information about your hormones. If you have PCOS, you might feel like you're on a roller coaster and that your body follows no pattern at all—that's okay. The important thing is just to record what you see.

Menstrual color: This can shift day to day or cycle to cycle. It indicates whether your blood is flowing at a healthy rate.

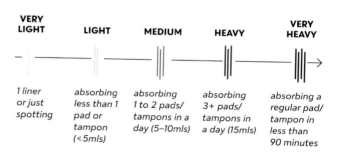

BRIGHT RED	DARK BROWN/RED	LIGHT PINK	DEEP PURPLE
Sign of healthy blood flowing at a normal rate	Sign of slow blood flow (oxidized blood) and low progesterone	Can be associated with low estrogen or high stress	Can indicate excess estrogen

Volume/weight: A completely normal period will progress either from days of light to heavy and back to a light flow, or it may start heavy and progressively lighten up.

VERY LIGHT	LIGHT	MEDIUM	HEAVY	VERY HEAVY
1 liner or just spotting	absorbing less than 1 pad or tampon (<5mls)	absorbing 1 to 2 pads/tampons in a day (5–10mls)	absorbing 3+ pads/tampons in a day (15mls)	absorbing a regular pad/tampon in less than 90 minutes

Cervical fluid: It's normal for your cervix to release fluid leading up to ovulation. The clearer, stretchier, smoother, and more lubricative it becomes, the more you are fertile and approaching ovulation. That is because sperm travel easily through this type of fluid, helping them to reach the fallopian tubes. In a "perfect" cycle, cervical mucus dries up and disappears after ovulation and won't return until after the next period.

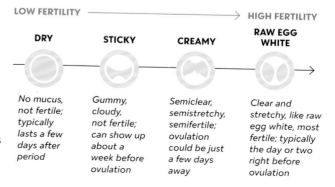

LOW FERTILITY → HIGH FERTILITY

DRY	STICKY	CREAMY	RAW EGG WHITE
No mucus, not fertile; typically lasts a few days after period	Gummy, cloudy, not fertile; can show up about a week before ovulation	Semiclear, semistretchy, semifertile; ovulation could be just a few days away	Clear and stretchy, like raw egg white, most fertile; typically the day or two right before ovulation

MOOD

I focus on when I feel happiest in the month, when I notice mood shifts, when I feel a lack of energy, and when my sex drive goes up or down. Being in touch with your mood changes can help you control your emotions as well as improve your mental health.

FOOD

Journaling also changed my eating habits. Take note of what you eat and of any symptoms that occur after eating. Your notes could show that every time you have a certain meal you crash and need coffee to stay awake. That's a helpful insight!

OTHER SYMPTOMS

Take note of any days you experience cramping, acne breakouts, breast tenderness, bloating, bowel irregularities, headaches, fatigue, nausea, sleep disturbances, and anything out of the ordinary.

It's also a good idea to note any days you have intercourse, as well as days you take medications.

INTERPRETING

Some signs you've kept an eye on while journaling can be directly attributed to progesterone or estrogen issues.

Estrogen dominance:

- Worse than normal PMS symptoms (breasts swelling, headaches, acne flare-ups, etc.)
- Heavy periods
- Bloating and weight gain
- Mood swings (quick and dramatic)
- Irritability (*everything* is getting under your skin)
- Decreased sex drive
- Hair loss
- Trouble sleeping
- Memory fog
- Hot flashes and night sweats

Low progesterone:

- Low sex drive
- Irregular or missed periods
- Breast tenderness
- Spotting between periods
- Vaginal dryness
- Hot flashes
- Depression or anxiety
- Sleep issues or insomnia
- Fatigue
- Memory fog
- High stress
- Water retention
- Weight gain

The main point is just to journal, no matter how. This gives you an objective way to view signs before and after any intervention to see if things are improved. For example, you may notice an improved symptom but also a new side effect from a medication. Your notes help you weigh the risk and reward.

SAMPLE JOURNAL

Look for an app or create your own template similar to this one to help you keep track of the many signs and symptoms listed on the previous spread.

	MAR 31 / S	1 / S	2 / M	3 / T	4 / W	5 / T	6 / F	7 / S	8 / S	9 / M	10 / T	11 / W	12 / T	13 / F	14 / S	15 / S
CYCLE DAY	**1**	**2**	**3**	**4**	**5**	**6**	**7**	**8**	**9**	**10**	**11**	**12**	**13**	**14**	**15**	**16**
CERVICAL MUCUS — CLEAR/STRETCHY													■	■	■	
CERVICAL MUCUS — CREAMY/EGG WHITE												■				
CERVICAL MUCUS — STICKY										■	■					
CERVICAL MUCUS — DRY		■														■
MENSTRUAL VOLUME	L	M	H	H	M	L	VL									
COLOR	B	BR	BR	BR	BR	B	B									
INTERCOURSE	X						X		X		X				X	X
CRAMPS	X	X										X		X		
BLOATING											X					
ACNE	X	X														
BREAST TENDERNESS	X															
BOWEL IRREGULARITY		X	X													
HEADACHE	X	X														
FATIGUE			X													
NAUSEA															X	
SLEEP DISTURBANCE	X									X						

NOTES

- Cycle day 1: *So relieved I got my period! Means that I'm not actually a crazy betch—just my hormones.*
- Cycle day 5: *Feeling energized to work out again.*
- Cycle day 7: *Went live on social media . . . like, who am I?*
- Cycle day 8: *My jokes were unhingeddddd today.*
- Cycle day 9: *Waking up and feeling motivated!*
- Cycle day 10: *Ordered Chinese. Immediate stomachache. Forgot to ask if menu items contained gluten.*
- Cycle day 14: *Super horny.*

Date	16	17	18	19	20	21	22	23	24	25	26	27	28	29	30	1	2	3
Day	M	T	W	T	F	S	S	M	T	W	T	F	S	S	M	T	W	T
Cycle day	**17**	**18**	**19**	**20**	**21**	**22**	**23**	**24**	**25**	**26**	**27**	**28**	**29**	**30**	**31**	**32**	**33**	**34**
	XX		X				X		X									
								X		X	X							
							X			X	X							
						X	X	X										
								X										
											X							
						X	X	X		X								
				X								X						

Notes:
- Cycle day 17: *Feeling extra grateful and happy today.*
- Cycle day 21: *Intense urge to color coordinate my closet.*
- Cycle day 23: *Crying my eyes out for no reason.*
- Cycle day 24: *Irritable. Everything Tom does pisses me off.*
- Cycle day 25: *Binge-eating snacks. Nothing will satisfy my hunger.*
- Cycle day 26: *Feeling overwhelmed. Breakouts around my chin. Want to feel normal again.*

Seeking Answers

My first misdiagnosis was in 2017 when I went to see a doctor for recurring migraines around the time of my period, as well as irregular cycles. My irregular cycle didn't seem to faze the doctor. She wrote it off as actually very common to miss a period or two and that my active lifestyle was probably causing it. Granted, I was exercising four to five days a week, but I was no Olympic athlete training several hours a day or pushing my body to extremes. I felt like she was quick to judge that I must be overexercising, which wasn't a thorough answer for me considering she didn't even ask about my lifestyle history. I felt like I was being blamed for trying to be healthy, but I had done no prior research of my own at this point, so I didn't know how to respond. She didn't seem concerned about my irregular cycle, so why should I be? We will talk about the importance of advocating for yourself and why it's important to understand your doctor's style and philosophy. I left the doctor's office that day with the simple notion that I was potentially exercising too aggressively; I went home to tell Tom that I was advised nothing was wrong or concerning with my cycle health.

Eventually we learned about PCOS and did enough of our own research that we wanted a doctor simply to confirm whether or not I had PCOS, and if so, to help manage the diagnosis.

FINDING THE RIGHT DOCTOR

The doctor-patient relationship in an ideal world is a two-way street—find someone who you can schedule a handful of appointments with per year, as well as a doctor whose philosophy on managing PCOS aligns with your own. For us, our favorite doctors are the ones who over-explain the why's to their thought processes: *"This is why your body feels this way." "This is why you are having these pains." "We might want to try this approach, and this is why."*

Questions you can ask your doctor:

- What criteria do you use to diagnose PCOS?

- How would you describe your approach to treating PCOS?

- What medications might you use for treatment that *aren't* hormonal birth control?

- Will you run labs and diagnostics, and what will those monitor/track?

- Do you routinely monitor markers, such as cholesterol, blood pressure, and diabetes?

- How often do you recommend we meet to take labs and discuss progress?

- Do you have recommendations for further resources I can consult on the topic of PCOS?

- Will you consider my goals in your treatment approach, whether that be optimizing fertility or regulating menstruation?
- Do you refer to specialists for any conditions?

NAVIGATING HORMONAL BIRTH CONTROL

Hormonal birth control certainly has its benefits. It can help with acne and painful periods, and it's convenient if you don't want to get pregnant. There are even studies out there showing a correlation between birth control and women's educational and economic advancements. It can take the form of the pill, skin patch, vaginal ring, and hormone-releasing contraceptive coils.

But potential side effects aren't always talked about. While you may be aware of some of the common ones (depression, weight gain, headaches, mood changes, and lower sex drive), it's also associated with an increased risk of autoimmune disease, heart attack, and thyroid and adrenal disorders. Another common effect is post-pill amenorrhea (your period not coming back after the pill), something very common in PCOS.

Too often, PCOS symptoms are swept under the rug by a blanket tendency to prescribe hormonal birth control rather than identifying the root cause. We truly believe the intention of the doctor is to help you feel better, but not all women are open to hormonal birth control for various reasons, and if you are trying to conceive, then it certainly isn't an option. Sometimes it feels as though the only thing a doctor can offer is birth control. You may be taking the pill for contraceptive reasons or a slew of other "female problems" that a doctor would throw the pill at. Keep in mind when being given the pill, it won't fix your period.

Here's how it works: "The pill" is essentially a synthetic estrogen and progesterone (or progesterone-only) pill that blocks the release of eggs from the ovaries, halting ovulation (in most cases). This means that the bleed you experience when you take the pill is not technically a period, which can only happen as the result of ovulation, which you're not doing. Your pill bleed is actually a withdrawal bleed, or your body's response to the sudden drop in your hormonal levels from the medication. So in short, your cycle symptoms may go away on the pill, but that's because you are not actually having a cycle at all.

This means that whatever problems you have *before* the pill will likely return when you get off the pill and your body starts trying to resume its cycle again. There are many risks and benefits to weigh. If you do have underlying issues and one day you want to address them or possibly start a family, keep in mind that the pill is like having a leak in a roof and putting a bucket under to collect the water, but never actually fixing the hole in the roof.

If you do decide to start or continue taking hormonal birth control, it's important to journal about your symptoms, as discussed earlier in the chapter. If you're coming off the pill, keep an eye out for post-pill amenorrhea, which means missing your period for more than 3 months if you were previously regular, or 6 months if you were irregular. Be sure to report back to your doctor if this is the case.

Make sure to inquire about treatments other than the pill that your doctor has tried and seen great success with: What does that treatment consist of? Does it fit in with your lifestyle? What are realistic results you can expect given how previous patients of your doctor have fared?

MEDICATIONS BEYOND THE PILL

Beyond taking the pill, there are two other categories of medicine typically used alongside lifestyle changes and diet to manage PCOS symptoms. These are great at jump-starting your journey but will not fix root causes, so make sure you talk to your doctor about an exit plan if you still have the intention of fixing the issues at a later time.

Antiandrogen therapies are drugs that block the effects of androgens (male hormones) in your body, such as testosterone. They can be used to slow down or minimize masculinizing effects of the male hormones. You might notice male-pattern hair growth or male-pattern balding, acne, and ovulation issues that are helped with these therapies.

Your doctor may recommend spironolactone or minoxidil. Minoxidil, more commonly known as Rogaine, is a medication that can be applied to the skin to help promote hair growth. It can be useful if you notice male-pattern baldness occuring due to excess androgens.

Spironolactone is a medication that can block the effects of androgens. Your provider may prescribe this to help manage symptoms like abnormal hair growth or acne. Keep an eye out for and start tracking any of these potencional side effects: low sex drive, depression, electrolyte deficiency, diarrhea, hot flashes, breast tenderness, and skin rash.

Medications to manage effects of insulin resistance can be important to treating your PCOS. These medications decrease the levels of circulating insulin and also reduce adipose (fat) tissue. Metformin is a diabetes-class medication often used for PCOS patients. Typically when you have a higher body mass index (BMI), doctors will recommend this treatment to jump-start weight loss and improve insulin sensitivity, which can lead to regaining ovulation.

Inositol and berberine are supplements you can find in several forms on the market. Patients who report unwanted side effects from metformin may benefit from one of these options, which offer similar blood sugar-lowering control.

Ditching the Pill

By age 14, my face was a nesting ground for cystic acne. It was the type of acne my friends and family would try to convince me wasn't noticeable, which didn't help my self-esteem. While my cheeks remained untouched of red boils and inflamed pustules, my chin and jawline were consumed with tens of hundreds of little fluid-filled bumps under the skin.
I felt dismissed when I would confide in people about this insecurity. It felt as though because my acne wasn't as prominent, covering the surface of my whole face, I should be grateful this was all I was getting with puberty.

This same dismissal would continue into my adult life before being diagnosed with PCOS when I would confide in those around me about my symptoms of irregular bloating. My family and friends would argue that "I was still skinny." I couldn't understand why the conversation always went back to physical appearance. Never once did it revolve around my health and wellness or was it taken into consideration that these signs and symptoms were my body trying to tell me something.

Let's focus on 16-year-old me who, after 2 years of countless acne facials and trying every acne solution in the book (which, yes, included Proactiv, the infamous acne-fighting solution deemed to solve all of our acne problems), I was finally taken to a dermatologist to see what they could do for me. Walking in, I knew birth control was a probable treatment because I had friends who were put on the pill for their acne—but I never knew why. What did this pill exactly do to make everyone's face so clear? At 16, no one expects you to advocate for yourself and ask questions. All I knew was birth control was marketed as the best for making acne disappear, and if I could get on the pill, I also wouldn't have to have the awkward conversation with my mom about whether or not I was having sex because, well, I was on the pill. And so it began. At the ripe age of 16, I started using the Band-Aid approach to my health by masking my symptoms instead of treating an underlying condition.

CHAPTER 3

A LIFESTYLE TO MANAGE YOUR DIAGNOSIS

RACHAEL: "Can PCOS go away?" **is something I'm sure you've asked yourself by this point. Hell, it was the first thing I Googled when I got my diagnosis. Although there is no cure for PCOS, your symptoms can be managed and you *can* start to feel like yourself again. For some of you, you're about to feel like an entirely new version of yourself—someone who has more energy, connection to your body, newfound happiness, and an appreciation for how your cycle operates. Learning how to manage my cycle was one of the most empowering things I have felt as a woman, and I'm excited to be able to share these tools with you to help nurture your body and rebalance your hormones.**

Self-care, as Tom would say, is a crucial ingredient to managing your PCOS. There are a multitude of hormonal changes, emotional changes, and physical changes that your body will experience during the menstrual cycle. We will touch on each of these topics as we navigate through the phases, along with tangible ways to hopefully inspire you to work with your body and not against it.

Throughout each phase, we will also equip you with types of movement that will support your PCOS and make you aware of types of movements that can be counterproductive to your healing. There are plenty of us who hate exercising but want to find a way to enjoy it. We want you to embrace an exercise routine, but don't beat yourself up when the routine changes. We are not saying you need to become a robot. Gosh, we have routines that last a week, some last months, and others we've done for years. The internal battle of fighting to keep a routine that your body is just not having is far more taxing than adjusting until you find that sweet spot. Every menstrual cycle for every individual will be different. Do what's best for you and your body, and remember this is a guide—not a mandate. Use these suggestions as inspiration for a starting point or simply a way to try something new. No matter what activities you choose to partake in, commit to doing them for yourself, and have some fun.

WELCOME TO THE
MENSTRUAL PHASE

What I used to hate most about being a woman is now sacred to me. Getting my period, or entering "shark week" as we call it in our house, no longer scares me. At this point in your cycle, your hormones are at their lowest. The drop in progesterone causes the uterus to contract and result in the shedding of the uterine lining, aka the bleed. I'll be honest, my period used to simply be the red or green light to knowing if I was pregnant or not, but now it is the indication to so many other health markers going on in my body. The absence of your period, the color, and even the amount you bleed can tell you about underlying imbalances. Be prepared to feel a little run down and sluggish at this point, and don't be afraid to match the energy in the room. Cater to your body's needs, but also don't use this time to become completely irresponsible to your body. I get it. When you feel like eating poorly, instead eat foods to nurture your body. You will feel so much better. The same goes for exercising! There's a yoga studio in Chicago called the Shiva Shack that I would attend during my menstrual phase, and I would take the 8 p.m. candlelight yin class. It was basically a nap for my mind. Soft, calming candles surrounded the room while we practiced light stretching to relieve stress and anxiety and alleviate pain. I even got Tom to participate. We were never more

relaxed going to bed. It's easy to forget just how important spending quality time with ourselves really is. Sometimes it's easier said than done—to put your life on hold to enjoy me-time—but I try to always make it a priority, even if for 20 minutes of that day. Remember: self-care isn't selfish.

MENSTRUAL MOVEMENTS

Every period is different, so do what you need to do to feel your best. If that means getting your exercise in by parking at the far end of the parking lot to get some extra steps, do it. Your naps are welcome here, too. Try these movements:

- Walking

- Stretching

- Breathing

- Yin yoga

- Rest

- Gardening

- Playing a musical instrument

- Geocaching (don't knock it till you try it)

WELCOME TO THE
FOLLICULAR PHASE

When you find me at my funniest on Instagram stories, it's because I've entered into the follicular phase. Now, I love and honor my body during every phase of the menstrual cycle for different reasons, but the follicular phase is unmatched. The rise of estrogen is happening, and my body knows it. My creative juices are flowing, and those other juices I produce are starting to get thick and sticky. You will notice your emotions soar to new levels of energetic and outgoing. The part I love the most is being fearless and stepping outside my comfort zone. It all comes more naturally during this phase. Mark this time on your calendar to be social and also to plan for what you want to accomplish for the weeks ahead. Let's be honest here. Mentally, you're not in the mood to produce your life's greatest work, but you are in the mood to strategize what that plan looks like and how you are going to execute it step by step.

FOLLICULAR MOVEMENTS

It's time to try something new! You just finished your bleed, which means you're like a snake who just shed its old skin. You're no longer feeling weighed down—you feel physically and mentally lighter than you have in weeks! Now you may be saying to yourself "Really, Rachael, you just compared us to a snake?" Yes, everyone, I did. Tom had one in college, and as coauthor, we have to respectfully include his interests. So go be the fearless snake we all know you are and attack that prey (your new exercise class, of course!). Try these movements:

- Rock climbing
- Rowing
- Cardio dance
- Trampoline workout
- Zumba
- Belly dancing

WELCOME TO THE
OVULATORY PHASE

After a year of journaling my emotions, I can confidently tell you when I ovulate, I feel most alive. During this peak window, there's a surge in estrogen triggering the release of the luteinizing hormone (LH) and the rise of testosterone. It's a beautiful combination of hormones that takes the fearless energy you felt in the follicular phase and combines it with an unspoken confidence. It's the pregnancy glow without the pregnancy. An intensified sex drive you've been craving all month followed by, yes, a wetness in your panties. Which circles back to a very important topic: understanding your cervical mucus is a great tool to help track your cycle (see *Cervical Fluid* on page 42). Because you are most fertile during this time, mucus should resemble raw egg whites. I remember growing up and thinking something was wrong with me because I would wipe and it would be clear and stretchy. Actually, let's backtrack a little bit. One time in seventh grade, I slammed on my bike brakes a little too hard and the seat felt like it paralyzed my coochie. Shortly after that, my body started transitioning into puberty and my discharge down there started changing. For years, I thought the new onset of cervical mucus indicated that I broke my vagina on my bike seat. I forever blamed that instance for all the residue that would appear in my undies. To bring it back to where we started, take this small window you have during these few days and embrace the way you feel. Use the confidence and clarity to try something new in the bedroom, or instead, ask your boss for that raise.

OVULATION MOVEMENTS

Bring on the intense workouts and the intense sex. I'll let you define *intense* for yourself. With estrogen and testosterone at peak levels, you've got the energy to burn, so get after it. Try these movements:

- Hiking
- Aerial yoga
- Hot yoga
- Kickboxing
- HIIT classes
- Spin classes
- Sex!

WELCOME TO THE
LUTEAL PHASE

I've learned to lean into how my body responds during this part of my cycle because as someone who is an extrovert, this season of my cycle brings out the introvert in me. After ovulation, there is a dip in estrogen and your progesterone levels reach their high. This is when I find myself starting to nest. You could say my social calendar and my downstairs both dry up. I feel no draw to make dinner plans with friends and instead I find myself wanting to stay home, clean my house, and work on routines. If you are a people-pleaser like me, you can tend to feel very overwhelmed during this part of your cycle. Saying no to things will feel like the greatest victory. When I started journaling, this was when I noted those premenstrual symptoms occurring. After several months of noting the hormonal shift that was happening, I could now anticipate that my body may experience irritability or mood swings and prepare for it rather than crying my eyes out for days, questioning what was wrong with me. Give yourself permission to slow down. You'll feel the shift happening in your body, so don't fight it. If you need our Hulu or Amazon Prime password because #relaxing, shoot Tom a DM.

LUTEAL MOVEMENTS

With the shift in your hormones throughout this phase, you will also notice a shift in your energy. What felt good for your body during the first half of your cycle might not be the case for the second half. That Barry's HIIT boot camp you felt good at a week ago may now sound worse than medieval torture. As the days progress, take a step back from the high-intensity workouts and focus on strength training. Low-intensity workouts are gentler on the body as you prepare for menstruation. Try these movements:

- Biking
- Stand-up paddle boarding
- Yoga
- Swimming
- Dancing
- Barre class

Road Map to a Workout Routine

Junior year of high school I joined track. I lasted two practices and one meet. Technically three practices, if you count the time we ran past my home and I snuck in and waited till they made the loop back and I "finished" with the front of the team. Next, I tried at-home workout videos. After only a week, I quickly learned that workouts were going to have to be outside the vicinity of my home because I half-assed every video and held myself to no accountability. Next I joined the gym. I still feel strongly about the statement I'm about to make, so don't get mad at me: walking on a treadmill seems a nuisance. I would rather walk outside instead of walking in place, staring at a blank wall for 30 minutes. I did find some satisfaction with weight training, watching the weight I could lift increase and my body become more lean, but it all felt so isolating and lonely to me. So I tried classes, and a lot of them, until I fell in love with Pure Barre. It wasn't love at first sight, but it had potential, and I knew if I gave myself 2 weeks to implement a routine, then this could really be something. Pure Barre has three different class formats ranging from low-impact resistance training to interval training, which helped me switch up my routine. Plus it checked all the boxes for what was going to motivate me. It was expensive, which meant I had to attend classes to get my money's worth. Working out in a group setting also pushed me because I wasn't going to let the teacher see me not trying. They also had no refunds on cancellations, so when I made the commitment to go in advance, there was no backing out. It was all the things I needed to be held accountable. Did the workouts also help strengthen my pelvic muscle resulting in stronger orgasms? Absolutely. The point is, find what works for you. When the pandemic hit and studios were closed, I learned to love walking. I now incorporate it into my routine every day because the best type of exercise is the type you do regularly.

SELF-CARE PRACTICES

Self-care practices are the rituals and routines that often take a back seat on the priority list. Instead of trying to *find* time to incorporate these practices into our daily lives, let's focus on *making* the time. Both vital to our mental and physical health, these practices can help us acquire peace, stability, and most importantly, a chance to reset.

Participating in the act of self-care shows a great appreciation and love for yourself. Don't be afraid to hold a high regard for your own well-being. You are not being selfish by taking care of your own needs. While it's important to be good to others, make sure in doing so you're not sacrificing your own well-being. Tom and I were watching a cooking show (what else is new), and they said this quote that I think holds truth here: "*Sometimes the best thing to do for yourself is to keep your side of the street clean instead of trying to fix everything.*"

 SLEEP

Do not ditch on the zzZzzzs. Sleep is one of the most important lifestyle modifications you can make during your PCOS journey. So many symptoms are associated with inadequate hours of rest, which includes increased blood pressure, inflammation, and weight gain, just to name a few. If insomnia is something you deal with (been there), creating a bedtime routine might benefit you:

- Take a warm bath.

- Four words: exercise for better sleep (i.e., get some movement in throughout the day).

- Buy those blackout curtains.

- Set the thermostat low.

- Stop mindlessly scrolling before bed, and let your brain unwind (unless you are watching my content—then carry on).

- Unwind with a book (you can't go wrong with a Colleen Hoover read).

- Use sleep sounds. My personal favorite is to ask Alexa to "play rain forest sounds." You can thank me later.

 JOURNAL

Journaling is my secret to life. It's my favorite avenue to help with problem solving, keeping things in perspective, and finding clarity. I keep a digital journal that I share with the world, and then I keep a few for me. Remember: journaling can be as simple as writing the date on a page and saying "Today I felt happy." Here are two different ways that I've practiced the art of journaling:

- **Goal Setting:** I struggled with journaling at first and then I found the book *This Year I Will. . .* by Tiffany Louise. It's a 52-week guided journal to achieve your goals. Once a week, I spend 5 to 10 minutes answering prompts that ask me to reflect on things that happened in the past week that were movement or growth toward my goals. You are asked if there are any small wins you can celebrate, along with any highs and lows you have experienced and where you can make room for improvements. I have three copies of this book if that tells you anything about my obsession with how it has helped me.

- **Gratitude**: To bring more focus to each day, I start with *Two-Minute Mornings,* a journal by Neil Pasricha. Each morning, I answer three simple sentences: (1) What I will let go of? (2) What am I grateful for? and (3) What will I focus on? Taking these few moments to set intention to my day and reflect on what I'm most grateful for makes me feel like I'm starting my day with a big W.

 ## MEDITATE

There are so many beautiful health benefits I've gained from meditation to help manage my PCOS, especially when it comes to managing anxiety and stress. I've tried to get into meditation practices for years, and nothing was quite working until I downloaded the Calm app. I love listening to The Daily Jay by Jay Shetty, usually on my walks or before I go to bed.

 ## GET OUTSIDE

Nature is truly healing to both the mind and body. Go for a walk, sit under a willow tree, set up a picnic in the park, or just be. Use nature as a means to both soothe and restore the body while recharging mentally and improving your physical well-being. Women with PCOS are also more likely to have a vitamin D deficiency, so get out and enjoy a little sunshine, but don't forget your SPF 30!

 ## USE A SKIN CARE ROUTINE

Feeding your skin from the outside in is also a great regimen to add to your mornings and evenings. Not only that, but I find it calming and soothing. Look to incorporate as many clean beauty brands as possible, formulated without harmful ingredients like artificial dyes, parabens (chemicals that can act like estrogen and disrupt normal hormone function) and phthalates (endocrine disrupters).

This is my nighttime routine in order of application: cleansing balm, cleanser, retinol serum, moisturizer, eye cream, and face oil. This is my morning routine in order of application: cleansing water, exfoliating (twice a week), hyaluronic acid serum, vitamin C serum, moisturizer, eye cream, and sunscreen.

 ## READ

Reading is a relaxation method to allow yourself a temporary escape from reality. Heighten the experience by cozying up with your favorite blanket and a warm beverage in a peaceful location. Joining a book club also offers a social experience, creating a sense of belonging. I love getting together with my club once a month. First, it's an incentive to actually read a book, but also red wine and hors d'oeuvres, anyone?

 ## TAKE BATHS

Next time you draw a bath, focus on encompassing all your senses for a full-body experience. Create a *visually* calming environment with candles, *listen* to your favorite soundtrack, *sip* on your favorite drink, *feel* the relaxation of the Epsom salts, and take in the *smells* of the essential oils you're immersed in.

 ## CREATE A ROUTINE

Routines create structure, and structure allows for more productive and positive days. Routines also help instill good habits even in times of unpredictability and stress. Try creating a morning routine to bring a sense of accomplishment to the start of your day. This can include setting an alarm, making your bed, stretching, implementing your skin care routine, drinking a glass of water, and journaling.

 ## LIMIT SOCIAL MEDIA

Limiting the amount of social media you consume can significantly reduce levels of anxiety and depression, improving your mental health. There's a "fear of missing out" or an all-consuming feeling that social media brings when we see what everyone else is doing, and we and feel as though our lives are not as satisfying. Remember, comparison is the thief of joy, so we must *stop comparing* and *start living*.

 ## GIVE BACK

There's a happiness that comes with giving rather than receiving, no matter how big or small the act. Whether you are donating your time, money, or skills, there are certain chemicals inside the brain that get released, creating what is known as the "giver's glow"— a sense of joy and peace. Word of caution: if your idea of giving back is feeding one college kid, be aware it could grow into a community of hundreds.

 ## REST

Rest looks different for everyone. We spend time in our day working, eating, walking the dog, and running errands, so why should rest be any different? Release the constant need to always be doing and let yourself just be. Regardless on how you choose to rest, use some of these self-care practices to slow down and realign with your mind and body.

 ## DRINK WATER

You've heard it before, but we're here to remind you again. Drink the water. It's the answer to everything. It's not hard. Water is ultra-refreshing and can be enhanced with lemon or fruit to add a little bit of taste. So stop complaining and drink the damn water!

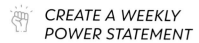 ## *CREATE A WEEKLY POWER STATEMENT*

A power statement is a clear affirmation that supports your values, character, and goals. On Sundays, I create or find a power statement that gets my mind and body ready for the week. Here are some of my past power statements:

> *Continue with confidence in all you do.*
>
> *Your presence is your power.*
>
> *Always be proud of yourself for showing up.*
>
> *Do one thing a day that scares you.*
>
> *Rome wasn't built in a day.*
>
> *Knowledge gives you power.*
>
> *Whatever you are not changing you are choosing.*

 ## *CONSIDER THERAPY*

Self-care is also about setting aside time to focus on matters we may not be able to tackle alone. Therapy is an intentional action to care for yourself and an investment in your mental health. Being able to explore your thoughts and feelings in a safe space is a beautiful way to inspire change and allow for self-awareness and self-exploration to make healthier choices in life—both in and out of the kitchen.

SUPPLEMENTS

Remember supplements are just that—supplemental. They are not replacements for a healthy diet, but they can definitely provide some much-needed help.

Keep in mind supplements are unregulated and not all created equal. Look for NSF or USP certifications. These are backed by research supporting the claims. Consider some of the following, and run them by your doctor:

- **L-theanine** is an amino acid that has a calming effect. It's good to help with kicking caffeine addiction.
- **Magnesium** helps with water retention and supports regular bowel movements.
- **Multivitamin** is intended to fill nutritional gaps. If trying to conceive, it's recommend to start taking prenatal vitamins—which contain more folic acid—3 months before you become pregnant.
- **Omega-3** encourages progesterone production and reduces inflammation.
- **Probiotics** helps with digestion and gut health. They can reduce inflammation and help regulate androgens and estrogen.
- **Vitamin B complex** is helpful for fighting off insulin resistance and supporting energy levels.
- **Vitamin C** promotes great blood and strong bones.

- **Vitamin D** is vital to your endocrine system. A deficiency is common in PCOS patients. It's linked to improved fertility and pregnancy outcomes and can help depression.

- **Vitamin E** is important for vision health, reproduction, and the health of your blood and skin.

- **Vitex (tincture or capsule)** boosts low progesterone levels.

- **Zinc** can boost fertility and help your immune system. It also helps with unwanted hair growth.

NATURAL REMEDIES

Natural medicine allows the body to heal through its own processes. Not only is the natural way, well, *natural,* but it's also more cost effective than medication, comes with little to no side effects, and is easier to obtain. Here are a few cheat-sheet remedies to include in your day to day:

- **Apple cider vinegar** relieves bloating, cramps, and PMS symptoms. Also, it regulates blood sugar levels.

- **Black cohosh** is an herb to support estrogen.

- **Cinnamon** is for blood sugar management, gut health, and anti-inflammatory properties.

- **Dandelion** supports liver detoxification.

- **Ginger** relieves muscle soreness and helps with digestion.

- **Holy basil** helps with blood sugar, weight gain, and cortisol levels.

- **Honey** is a natural anti-inflammatory and antioxidant.

- **Kefir** aids in digestion.

- **Milk thistle** detoxifies hormonal buildup.

- **MUD/WTR** is an adaptogenic coffee alternative with a fraction of the caffeine.

- **Peppermint** relieves bloating.

- **Tart cherry juice** lowers inflammation.

- **Tea** There are far too many and too many benefits! This is a good search-and-find-what-you-need category.

- **Turmeric (or curcumin)** suppresses inflammatory chemicals, helps with gut health, and decreases insulin resistance.

HOUSE SWAPS

PCOS is one of the most common endocrine disorders in women. Endocrine disrupters are harmful chemicals that act as synthetic hormones disrupting your system. Exposure to these endocrine-disrupting chemicals (EDCs) can happen anywhere from consumer products to the water we drink, to the air we breathe. These household swaps are simple changes to reduce the toxins we absorb and minimize the burden on our bodies in our everyday environments:

- **Plastic food containers can have harmful chemicals.** Make sure any plastic you use is BPA free or swap for glass or for another reusable option, like silicone bags.

- **Invest in clean personal care.** Makeup, hair products, skincare products, perfume, and sunscreen can all contain harmful ingredients. Luckily, there are so many nontoxic alternatives. Clean products won't contain ingredients like parabens, formaldehyde, synthetic fragrances, phthalates, and oxybenzone, among many others that can disrupt your hormones and overload your liver.

- **Cleaning products and air fresheners can also be filled with synthetics and chemicals.** Our favorite nontoxic cleaning brand is Branch Basics for cleaning products and detergents. Not only are the products simple, gentle, and effective, but one of the founders, Allison Evans, was diagnosed with PCOS, inspiring her to toss the toxins and help empower others to create an environment in which their families can thrive.

- **Clean up your cookware.** Opt for stainless steel, cast iron, or ceramic instead of traditional nonstick cookware. We also stopped using aluminum foil and swapped in parchment paper. The research shows that the minimal amount of aluminum that would leach into your food isn't harmful, but we like to do easy little swaps to lighten the toxic load.

- **Tampon alternatives come in all shapes and sizes.** Your vaginal wall is directly exposed to chemicals from your tampons where the toxins can enter your bloodstream. Just as concerned as we are about the additives in our food, tampons may be loaded with dyes, fragrances, and pesticides. Be on the lookout for organic tampons or pads. Good alternatives to tampons include menstrual cups, discs, period underwear, and even sponges. I really enjoyed the brand Saalt for a menstrual cup and found after a few applications of trial and error it was not as scary as I thought it would be.

FOOD

One of the most important self-care practices you can focus on is the foods you put in your body. We believe what goes in the body dictates so much of how we feel that we've dedicated an entire part of the book to it. Onward to Part 2, and how food impacts our bodies.

A Tampon Chronicle

I was now 6 months into my journey of womanhood and about to spend the entire summer at my family's lake house in Indiana. Avoiding the beach wasn't an option, and I knew my maxi pad wouldn't cut it. It was time. The day of self-exploration was closing in on me, a crippling anxiety that consumed me when I thought about tampons. It wasn't a question of what if it gets stuck; it was simple in my mind . . . the string will break, and this will get lost inside of me. I was not entering this endeavor of inserting a tampon alone. No; I recruited my older cousin to simply insert it for me. We purchased the smallest-size tampon on the market, a "slim," suitable for first timers experimenting with period products. The application went better than expected. With no shame, I had a seasoned vet by my side to glide it in for me. We left the bathroom that afternoon with sight of a visible string right where it should be—success.

You would think I just lost my virginity by the pride that consumed me. I did it. The confidence was soaring. After several hours though, my mother introduced a new fear to me known as toxic shock syndrome, which by the name led my imagination to believe that my body would start seizing if the tampon stayed too long inside of me. Back in the bathroom at my lake house after a day of swimming, I sat on the toilet and tried to pull it out. Nothing. It wasn't budging. You're absolutely kidding me. The string was there, but something was forbidding it from moving. I called in reinforcements, and I knew it was bad when my cousin attempted to pull it out and I watched her eyes fill with fear and worry.

"911, what's your emergency?" were those fatal last words I heard before my mom took the call off speaker phone and this imaginary fear I had of getting a tampon stuck was a reality. The scene was a sight to see. I was laying naked in the bathtub with my legs spread-eagle while my mom was reporting what she saw to the dispatcher and my cousin was holding my hand. The next moment happened quickly, as they were instructed to cover my eyes with a cloth, and that's when I saw it: a 10-inch butcher knife. Before I could panic, I felt an immense release and the tampon went soaring. Turns out that fateful day my mom had to use the knife to "pop my cherry"—a thin layer of skin from my hymen was blocking the exit for the tampon to be released. But it didn't hurt . . . really.

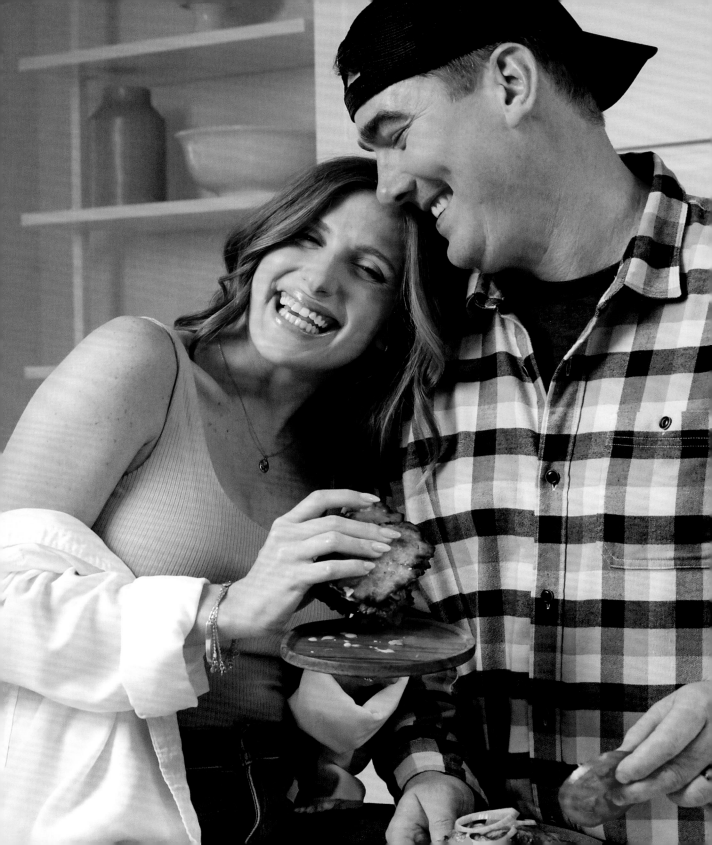

PART 2

THE MEALS SHE ATE

We've learned there's not a one-size-fits-all "diet" for PCOS. This will be a very individualized journey for each of you. What is right for one person may not work for another. Whether you're dealing with chronic low-grade inflammation, insulin resistance, a gut imbalance, or stress and adrenal dysfunctions, food can provide natural healing to the body. This section of the book will introduce our approach to food along with staples, techniques, and recipes to support each phase of your cycle.

Each phase has a list of foods that are here to help in a number of practical and medicinal ways. Some foods activate the metabolism, some generate warmth in the body, some help your liver metabolize estrogen, and so on. Each list is comprised of unprocessed, real foods filled with micronutrients that will support your overall health. We love that these lists take out the dreaded "what's for dinner?" question because now you will have a reference guide to consult when grocery shopping and planning out your meals. We want to reiterate that this is a guide, not a rule book. While these foods are listed in specific phases, you can absolutely overlap them.

Lastly, it's an honor to share our recipes with you. You often hear people talk about the love and care that goes into a recipe. We think of the handwritten recipe cards handed down through a family. When you care about and love the people you are cooking for, you pour your heart into the food. When you're measuring, smelling, and tasting a recipe along the way, it truly tastes like home and becomes a moment in your shared history with the people you're serving.

I (Tom) recently asked my mom for some of my favorite recipes from growing up. She responded that they are simple and kind of boring. It hit me then that the reason I can close my eyes and taste the dish is not because it's revolutionary, but because no one would be able to recreate it perfectly except my mom, who created it for me with love. When cooking, make these recipes your own, and don't get caught up in exact measurements or minor "flaws." I have zero professional cooking training. I do it because it gives me joy, helps my wife, and puts smiles on hundreds of college students' faces, and now I am lucky enough to share it with you all. As you cook, the most important ingredient will always be remembering the why—giving yourself to others is the true joy.

CHAPTER 4

OUR APPROACH TO FOOD

TOM: Our food journey started when we did a Whole30 elimination diet. You can read more in our introduction on pages 19 and 20. Ever since we got married in 2017, we have been on a quest to evaluate how the foods we eat impact our health and how Rachael can mitigate the symptoms of PCOS with thoughtful nutrition. In short, we know that a nutrient-dense diet, which strategically emphasizes *real foods,* certain nutrients during certain phases of the cycle, and also avoids gluten, dairy, added sugars, and other inflammatory ingredients is the strongest approach.

YOUR NEW "DIET"

Your eating habits need to become a *lifestyle* and not a crash-course diet because PCOS (among other disorders like celiac disease and endometriosis) doesn't have a cure, so you're in this for the long haul. Our goal in this chapter is to introduce you to topics that will jump-start your new lifestyle and give you a better understanding of how and why we approach food the way we do. Each of these topics could have their own books—and they do! (Not written by us, of course.) But hopefully this chapter provides you with enough information to inspire you to do more research and gain a deeper understanding of how different types of foods affect our bodies.

Even if you don't have a disorder, focusing on real foods and these principles can be beneficial to everybody. Remember, we are working on bringing balance back to our hormones. For women with PCOS, the idea that pain and discomfort are "just a part of womanhood" is beyond ridiculous. You have the power to choose the foods that can influence everything in your body for better or for worse: your period, PMS, pain, cramps, acne, and more.

One of the first approaches we take to mitigate these symptoms is to eliminate the amount of inflammatory foods we consume and incorporate as many anti-inflammatory foods as possible. This will promote a healthy gut with good bacteria, balanced stomach acid, and a strong and healthy lining.

We also avoid two foods known to disrupt hormones: dairy and soy. Your hormones are already out of sync with PCOS, so we limit our intake of foods that can further disrupt these hormones.

Food is not simply what you eat but also how you *absorb* it. Have you ever looked down in the toilet and seen full corn kernels in your stool? Because I remember the first time that happened to me and thinking "*Well, shit . . . what happened that this didn't digest properly?*" It's important to support the digestive process and allow your body to break down nutrients in order for you to be able to absorb them. We do this by intentionally preparing our foods in certain ways (more on this in the recipe chapters), but also with some tactics to support digestion directly. Some easy ways to do this are to stay hydrated, consume plenty of fiber, add apple cider vinegar to warm water after eating, use digestive bitters, and even take a couple extra chews before swallowing.

REAL FOOD

Throughout this book, we will often refer to the phrase *real food* as an easy way to summarize what you should focus on the most. Our favorite definition of real food is by Lily Nichols in her book *Real Food For Pregnancy*: "In a nutshell, real food is made with simple ingredients that are as close to nature as possible and not processed in a way that removes nutrients."

We want you to focus on eating food that hasn't been messed with—meaning it's as minimally processed as possible. Fruits, vegetables, animal proteins, herbs, and healthy fats are examples of real foods. Real food also means prioritizing how the food naturally grows. We look for these types of words when buying our food: organic, grass-fed, pasture-raised, heritage, and nongenetically modified (non-GMO). Try to find fruits and veggies that are in season and have been kept away from pesticides. Look for beef from cows that naturally grazed on grass in the open, not in confinement eating grains.

The quality of our food really does play a significant role in not only how the body absorbs and digests the food but also the level of satisfaction that comes from eating food that contains more vitamins and minerals. Take eggs, for example. Pasture-raised eggs—meaning the chickens got to roam, exercise, and eat a diet of grass and bugs that is natural to them—have significantly more nutrition than conventional eggs. There is research that they contain nearly twice as much omega-3 fatty acids, three times more vitamin D, four times more vitamin E, and seven times more beta-carotene. Can you see where two pasture-raised eggs for breakfast would be more satiating than four conventional eggs? When we started eating real food, the amount of food we ate dropped significantly.

By changing the types of food Rachael was consuming and preparing them in coordination with when her body both craved them and how her body was best able to absorb them, Rachael saw issues like hormonal acne, heavy menstrual bleeding, debilitating cramps, mood swings, and "missed" periods all disappear over just 3 months. Looking back and thinking this transition only took 3 months to accomplish is incredible, but during the process, 3 months without results at times felt daunting.

FOODS TO AVOID

These are the inflammatory and hormone-disrupting culprits we like to avoid in our diets.

TOP INFLAMMATORY FOODS

GLUTEN

For many people, eating gluten-containing foods aggravates the GI tract, which can cause the gut lining to become permeable, allowing toxins to freely flow into the bloodstream (called *leaky gut*). When this happens, it triggers the immune system to increase inflammation, which worsens PCOS symptoms.

ADDED SUGARS (SUCH AS SUCROSE AND HIGH-FRUCTOSE CORN SYRUP)

Once the body hits its limit of sugar that it can process, the body triggers an immune response. This also leads to insulin resistance and weight gain. The lesser amounts of fructose (a type of sugar) found naturally in fruits and vegetables and accompanied by fiber aren't the problem. It's added sugars often found in products such as dairy-free milk, ketchup, sauces, yogurts, etc. that promote inflammation.

REFINED VEGETABLE AND SEED OILS

Oils that have been processed at very high heats or with toxic solvents are more shelf stable, but the processing oxidizes the oil and can trigger inflammation in your body when you consume them. You'll find these harmful oils in fast food, margarines, and most of the processed foods at the grocery store. Instead of oils such as canola, vegetable, soybean, or sunflower, opt for less-refined, cold-pressed oils, such as olive, avocado, or coconut.

PROCESSED MEATS

Unfortunately, when many meats are processed, there are typically chemicals added to help preserve them. You might find these in lower-quality deli meats, sausages, bacon, and other cured meats. Highly processed animal products also contain advanced-glycation end products (AGEs), which are harmful compounds that are formed when protein or fat combine with sugar. AGEs trigger inflammation.

ALCOHOL

While moderate consumption of alcohol actually may have some benefits, overconsumption can lead to issues. Specifically looking at inflammation, heavy drinking can cause leaky gut and drive widespread inflammation.

REFINED CARBOHYDRATES

Carbs are not your enemy. Complex carbs make up a huge majority of our food list. It's the simple carbs or processed carbs that specifically drive inflammation. In processed carbs, the fiber is removed and the food is basically stripped of nutritional value. When your body breaks them down, they become sugar, triggering an immune response and leading to inflammation.

COMPLEX VS. SIMPLE CARBOHYDRATES

COMPLEX CARBOHYDRATES (digest slowly; found in their natural state)	SIMPLE CARBOHYDRATES (digest quickly; often contain refined sugar)
Fruits	Candy
Leafy greens and veggies	Soda
Starchy veggies (sweet potatoes, white potatoes, squashes)	Pastries (donuts, scones, croissants)
Beans, lentils, peas	Sugary cereals
Whole grains (brown rice, quinoa, oats)	White rice
Corn	White flour pasta
Pasta made from 100% brown rice, lentils, corn, quinoa, beans, nuts, and chickpeas	White breads
High in fiber *High in water* *High in antioxidants* *High in minerals* *High in vitamins* *Minimally processed*	*Low in fiber* *Low in minerals* *Low in vitamins* *Highly processed*

TOP HORMONE-DISRUPTING FOODS

SOY

Specifically in processed soy, there are compounds called *phytoestrogens* that behave similarly to estrogen. They have been shown to bind and block estrogen receptors. While the overall research on this can be mixed, there is enough out there that makes us want to avoid anything that can directly interfere with estrogen and exacerbate PCOS symptoms.

DAIRY

Dairy can get very confusing when it comes to whether it's good or bad for someone with PCOS—research points at connections rather than explicitly blaming the food. Dairy has been linked to causing hormonal acne, estrogen issues, inflammation, and even infertility. Some evidence suggests the quantity of dairy consumed is what's most significant. Rachael removed dairy from her diet to see if it would improve her hormonal acne, and she quickly noticed during the process that when removing it she had improved digestion also. Though more solid research is needed, there's enough to suggest a plethora of issues, so we chose to eliminate dairy from our diets.

THE DEAL WITH GLUTEN

Gluten is the name for a group of proteins found in grains, such as wheat, barley, and rye. (It's what gives gluten-containing foods their elastic-and-spongy texture.) Issues with digesting gluten exist on a spectrum. You might have a sensitivity, meaning you feel side effects and experience inflammation from consuming gluten, but perhaps it's not permanently damaging to your body. Then there is the autoimmune condition celiac disease, in which the body recognizes gluten as an invader and acts out against it. When this happens, the body's ability to absorb nutrients is permanently compromised. To make matters more confusing, you could also have a wheat allergy in which the body launches an attack against wheat, producing antibodies. It results in rashes, nausea, or other classic allergic reactions.

Women with PCOS may be more prone to gluten sensitivity and will benefit from a gluten-free diet. Gluten's proteins can disrupt gut health, spike insulin levels, and cause inflammation resulting in leaky gut and immune reactions.

It's well documented that in other countries outside of the United States, different wheat is used (soft wheat), which is lower in gluten, so the food may not affect the body the same way. Rachael's been dying to go to Italy to try the pizzas, pastas, and breads to test this theory out for herself. For now, here are some pointers for eliminating gluten from your diet.

1. **Know which grains are gluten-free,** and learn creative ways to enjoy your favorites. Quinoa, brown rice, millet, buckwheat, and oats are some of the more common gluten-free grains. By contrast, wheat, semolina, barley, rye, malt, and spelt do contain gluten. (As a side note, although oats are naturally gluten-free, they are often grown next to or processed in a facility with gluten-containing grains, leading to cross contamination. If you do notice an oat sensitivity, that may be why.) Refer to our swap lists (starting on page 93) to see other gluten substitutes.

2. **Know which common prepared foods contain gluten.** Cereal, cakes, cookies, crackers, pretzels, pasta, pizza crust, bread, and flour tortillas are more obvious culprits. Some less obvious offenders might be processed meats, fried foods, baking mixes, broths, soups (both creamy and clear), protein bars, granola, soy sauce, imitation crab, candy, dressings, marinades, beer, seasonings, vitamins, chips, restaurant eggs (some add pancake batter to thicken omelets and scrambled eggs), specialty mustards, taco seasoning, and ice cream, to name a few! You gotta learn to read those labels.

3. **Look for gluten-free certification labels.** It's worth noting that some products are able to carry this label while containing a small fraction (less than 20 parts per million) of gluten, but many will find that this small exposure is inconsequential. We go into more details on reading labels later, but this is a good start.

4. **Eat more produce!** Fruits and vegetables are naturally gluten free. We always have a bowl of cut-up fruit in the fridge to start the week, with clear plastic wrap covering it so it jumps out at us when we're grazing. Some of our favorite traditional bread swaps use produce, including the jibarito sandwich using plantains (page 166) and our version of the smash burger (page 165) using lettuce wraps.

5. **Clean out the pantry.** If your entire household isn't gluten-free, then make a gluten-free shelf or cupboard and stick to it. The next chapter is all about how to swap out foods.

6. **Be aware of beverages that contain gluten.** Since we mainly focus on foods, sometimes the liquids slip through the cracks. Some common beverages to be on the lookout for include beer, premade smoothies, and premade protein shakes.

THE DEAL WITH CAFFEINE AND ALCOHOL

Caffeine in general has pros and cons. It has been shown to improve alertness, contain antioxidants, boost your metabolic rate, and even lower your risk of type 2 diabetes. On the other hand, caffeine can disrupt your ability to fall asleep or prevent you from sleeping long enough, and we know sleep is essential to hormone function. PCOS gives our hormones enough trouble as it is. In addition to how it affects your sleep, caffeine can also raise your cortisol, a stress hormone that is typically already elevated in PCOS patients. This rise in cortisol leads to overeating and stress eating.

Listen, we get it. Who doesn't look forward to a morning cup of coffee? If you don't want to eliminate it completely, try to stick to moderation when it comes to caffeine. Before Rachael made the decision for herself to cut caffeine completely, she found a lot of success drinking matcha because it offered many other health benefits and had a lower caffeine content.

Like caffeine, alcohol also has pros and cons, so consumption in moderation is key. If you have PCOS and are taking metformin, consult your doctor and be cautious about mixing alcohol and medication. Alcohol can also produce high levels of insulin and drops in blood sugar, resulting in a number of health issues. If you or your doctor feel it's best to cut back on your alcohol intake to gain better control over your symptoms, then do so by all means. If you're reading this in hopes to gain a few tips on alcohol consumption and PCOS, here are some suggestions: Limit the amount of sugary drinks and mixers you are consuming. There may be a margarita on a summer day calling your name, but instead of having a frozen pitcher of lime slushie filled with sugar that will turn your tummy, swap out the frozen margarita for one on the rocks using fresh ingredients like agave and lime juice.

BALANCED BLOOD SUGAR

We want our blood sugar to stay **stable**. Extreme diets can take your blood sugar for a wild ride. Going for long periods of time without eating (fasting) can cause your blood sugar to drop, triggering sugar cravings.

You are not doing your body any favors by missing a meal. In fact, you are doing the exact opposite. The more frequently your blood sugar dips, the more often and intense your cravings can be, resulting in the worsening of insulin resistance. Similar to this, certain foods and combinations of foods (carbs, especially when eaten without protein or with processed sugars) can cause a spike in blood sugar. The spike often ends up being a crash later (going too low, too fast), which causes low energy, fatigue, and brain fog.

EAT ACCORDING TO YOUR CYCLE

Your body will never be in the same hormonal state twice in a month, so why should how you nourish your body be unchanging? In the next chapters, we are going to teach you how to feed your body in a way that will mimic your ever-changing shift in hormones and create optimal function in your cycle.

Probably one of the most common questions we get asked is, "I want to get started eating for my cycle, but I'm not regular or don't have a period at all. What phase should I start eating from?" Until your cycle is restored, skip our recommendations for the menstrual phase and start with the follicular phase for meal planning, shopping lists, and exercise. From there, let's pretend you have a very average 28-day cycle. After transitioning out of the follicular phase, you will continue eating based on that "healthy" cycle: Spend the first 8 days eating for the follicular phase, 3 days eating for the ovulatory phase, 12 days eating for the luteal phase, and finally 5 days eating for the menstrual phase. If at any time during this you begin your period, *congrats!* Take a moment to reflect and let that sink in: you've decided to take charge of your health, and this, my friend, is a victory! Once you begin to menstruate, jump right into the menstrual-phase foods. If your period does not restore after one cycle, continue the cycle again. Remember, this is not an exact science. Be kind and patient with yourself as you learn your body's natural rhythms over time.

TRUSTING YOUR BODY

As we shift our mindsets from a nondieting approach to cultivating a healthy relationship with real food, we want you to embrace listening to your body and eating what feels right for you. Throughout this book, that's exactly what we're doing: putting into words what listening to our bodies has taught us. Instead of approaching this lifestyle as a set of rules or restrictions, we want your food decisions to come from a place of self-care. Rachael has found that by nurturing a better relationship with her body, she now respects her body enough to know that certain foods don't serve her. Your body will communicate with you and tell you what's going on. The more you listen and learn from your body, the closer you will be to healing the root causes of many PCOS symptoms.

LEARNING TO SHOP

It's time to take a field trip to one of my favorite places in the world: the grocery store. We want to focus on keeping your shopping list to as many natural ingredients as possible. An easy way to approach the grocery store with this mentality is walking the perimeter of the store where perishable foods can be found: fresh fruit, veggies, and proteins. Then work your way into the aisles for your pantry staples and freezer goods: nuts, seeds, grains, canned goods, condiments, frozen fruit, frozen veggies, and frozen protein. Come prepared with a list so you don't impulse buy or become swindled by fancy packaging. (Rachael is a sucker for beautiful marketing.) And whatever you do, don't shop hungry.

If you're lucky enough to have access to a grocery delivery service, you can fill your cart online without having to leave home. Some grocery services deliver discounted items that have been rejected from the grocery store, usually because the produce is "ugly" or there was a surplus. We love options like this.

READING LABELS

Just because a food is labeled as gluten-free or dairy-free doesn't mean it's suddenly "healthy" for you. When Tom found out his beloved Oreos were launching a gluten-free edition, he went through a roller coaster ride of emotions. It started with excitement followed by the smack of reality that although they were gluten-free, Oreos still contain a laundry list of artificial ingredients. Lots of packaged foods have additives to maintain color and preserve shelf life. What we are looking for on labels are the ingredients: Are they real, and are they quality? Are there words we don't know? Hell, if we can't pronounce it, then we're probably not buying it. As obvious as this sounds, check for the gluten-free label. One of the first things we look for when reading a label is the tagline "contains" or "may contain" after the ingredients list. Here you might find listed sources of gluten. We also keep an eye out for sneaky names listed as added sugars. One ingredient you may find deceiving is natural flavors. The FDA at this moment doesn't require food labels to say what's in their "natural flavor" unless it includes a natural allergen. Although they may come from natural sources such as plants or animals, they are modified to enhance the flavors of food, not to add nutritional value. Here are some of the ingredients we avoid.

- **Sugar:** sucrose, dextrose, and high-fructose corn syrup.

- **Gluten:** wheat, rye, and barley.

- **Natural and artificial flavors**

- **Sulfites:** which preserves foods but can cause inflammation and allergies. Naturally occurring sulfites might be less harmful.

- **Carrageenan:** used to thicken foods and is often found in processed meats or dairy-free milks and causes inflammation.

OUR SHOPPING LIST

This is more than just a shopping list. These are our staple items that we carry in the house at all times. Every item on this list is foundational to recipes in each of the phases. Keep in mind that the goal isn't to only eat what is in the phase, but rather to incorporate those foods as staples within a wide nutrient-dense diet.

Produce

Avocado

Banana

Bell pepper

Carrot

Cucumber

Leafy greens (mixed, romaine, arugula, kale, or spinach)

Red onion

Strawberries or blueberries

Sweet potato or red potato

Two or three of the following: brussels sprouts, asparagus, green beans, beets, mushrooms, broccoli, or cauliflower

Refrigerated or frozen

Bacon (sugar-free with no preservatives)

Chicken (We always have frozen chicken—quarters, tenders, breasts—whatever is on sale.)

Dairy-free milk

Eggs

Frozen bag of vegetables (They have more nutrients than canned varieties. Just make sure you buy only vegetables—no sauces added.)

Frozen cauliflower pizza crust

Frozen fruit for smoothies (blueberries, bananas, strawberries, and raspberries)

Gluten-free bread or bagels (usually frozen)

Ground beef or turkey, lean (We always have at least a pound.)

Salmon (Fresh, if the full fillets are on sale, but we like to have some frozen on hand, too.)

Pantry and other

Apple cider vinegar

Almond or cashew butter

Avocado oil

Bone broth (high quality)

Chickpeas

Coconut aminos

Dijon mustard

Dried dates and other dried fruits

Extra-virgin olive oil

Fresh peppercorns (I will always love freshly cracked pepper lightyears more than already cracked.)

Gluten-free pasta

Grains: quinoa, brown rice, and lentils

Honey or agave syrup

Mayonnaise (high quality)

Nuts: almonds, walnuts, and pistachios

Protein bars (high quality)

Sea salt and kosher salt

Seeds: flax, chia, pumpkin, and sunflower

Tahini

STAYING ON TRACK

We found there are three common scenarios that open the door for breaking your positive new eating habits. Not to worry—we have strategies for combating them.

1. **You are starving and have nothing prepared, thawed, already made, or in mind. You need something quick!**

   When this happens, we know the staples from our shopping list are always on hand, so a salad is a viable option. Some of our favorite toppings include sunflower seeds, hard-boiled eggs, red onions, avocado, a protein, chickpeas, cucumber, and shredded carrots. Find our easy homemade dressings on page 102.

   Now, Rachael and I are not the type of people who can eat the same meals over and over, so we need options other than salads. For breakfast, we have our go-to quick meals: dairy-free yogurt with all the fixings that Rachael is craving, especially an add-in or two from the phase list (see page 103). We always have gluten-free bread on hand to quickly top with some nut butter or use for avocado toast. We enjoy grain-free cereal with some almond milk. And let's be honest, eggs take under ten minutes to make.

   Apple nachos are a simple snack that are also nutritious and super filling. Start by slicing your apple with an apple corer and toss them on a plate as your "chips." Drizzle your favorite nut butter over them, and sprinkle your favorite nuts and seeds or maybe even some coconut flakes on top.

   Rachael's favorite dinner in a pinch is microwaving a sweet potato. Her technique is to fill the bottom of a bowl with water and then spend several minutes poking holes in the sweet potato with a fork before placing it over the bowl to steam. She says poking the holes allows for the steam to escape so the sweet potato doesn't explode in our microwave, and since that hasn't happened yet, her technique is obviously flawless. She also doesn't shy on the toppings, ranging from sweet to savory.

   When we do plan ahead of time and meal prep, we have learned to always have a "salad" prepared, whether this be a chicken salad, potato salad, or coleslaw (which we consider a salad). These are nice to have as a snack or use as a side dish, especially ones that hold up well in the fridge.

   Outside of salads, you can often find these foods in our fridge to incorporate into meals in a pinch: homemade hummus, grilled chicken, and smoked salmon.

2. **You are traveling for work, vacation, a road trip, or any other reason you might be away from home for some time.**

   For our first 8 years together including 4 years of marriage, Rachael was a flight attendant, and I was in medical sales. We never had a -day period when we slept under the same roof. There was lots of travel both for work and fun, which also meant meal planning.

We always have a go-to snack for when the hunger kicks in and we need that emergency quick fix. For us, it's a clean-ingredient protein bar (such as RXBAR) and pistachios. Anytime we are traveling or even just running errands, a protein bar is coming with us. When Rachael is switching her purse or jacket, there is no doubt a protein bar or two will be making the switch as well.

Just like planning the trip, you need to have a plan for your meals, not just the snacks. For road trips, work trips, and airplanes, we bring our own food. (Yes, you can bring food through security at the airport . . . just not into other countries.) We typically pack a cooler on long road trips or work trips stored with sandwiches, fruit, jerky, hummus and vegetables, and grilled chicken tenders with honey mustard.

Rachael's experience as a flight attendant has given us a crash course on navigating airport foods, to which she reports back that the pickings are slim to none or cost $25 for a bed of wilted lettuce. Because of this, when traveling on an airplane, we always bring something, even if that's just a simple nut butter and jelly sandwich.

When we are on vacation, we make it a point to have a meal we cook ourselves. We enjoy going out to eat, but after 3 days of breakfast, lunch, and dinner out, not only is it difficult to manage, but it also loses its appeal. We love to stay in hotels or rentals with kitchenettes, and you better believe we're grocery shopping on day one.

When we're traveling in an unfamiliar area and find ourselves hungry, we seek out the following types of restaurants because they have more options for us:

- Mediterranean/Greek restaurants
- Middle Eastern restaurants
- Family-friendly or chain restaurants (such as Applebee's, Olive Garden, Chili's, and Cracker Barrel)
- Steakhouses
- Seafood restaurants
- Japanese restaurants

These are some fast food restaurants we like to go to because they incorporate real foods into their menu or have minimally processed and gluten-free options include:

- **Chipotle:** Salad bowl with romaine lettuce; black beans; carnitas, chicken, or carne asada; fajita veggies; fresh tomato, tomatillo-red chili, and/or tomatillo-green chili salsa; and guacamole
- **Five Guys:** A burger or double burger patty with lettuce bun, tomatoes, lettuce, pickles, mustard, and onion

- **Panera:** Fuji apple salad without cheese
- **Cava:** Salad greens with harissa, hummus, half harissa honey chicken and half roasted seasonal veggies, cabbage slaw, tomato and onion, diced cucumbers, pickled onions, fire-roasted corn, and lemon herb tahini dressing

Now here's our official thank you to restaurant owners, GMs, chefs, and staff. Because of you, the restaurant industry has come a long way with creating dishes that accommodate dietary restrictions. If you need to, never be ashamed to make a quick phone call to ask the restaurant about menu options. When you come across that unsuspecting place that can make a delicious meal while also being nutritious and accommodating to your dietary restrictions, make sure you take the time to support them. Post about it. Share it on social media. Write a Yelp review. That way, when others are Googling where they can eat, we as a community are able to make these places stand out.

3. **You are eating at a friend's house, dinner party, holiday family event, barbecue, or any other social event.**

We want to share our approach that we learned after much trial and error. First, we have to address the most brutal part: the judgment. This is not some fad diet! We are literally keeping Rachael healthy! We feel like we need to scream that sometimes when brushing up against ridicule. There is nothing worse than the feeling of saying you only eat gluten-free and receiving the look of scorn. You are not alone (and yes, it has pissed us off, too). This response sometimes takes the most amount of our patience, energy, and—honestly—kindness. Sharing that PCOS is a real diagnosis has helped us the most in this situation. Managing stress, reducing sugar, getting your workout in, and watching every ingredient you put into your body can be overwhelming. When you can share that you have PCOS and that certain foods noticeably change how you look, feel, sleep, and menstruate, then people will understand that the food you eat is your medicine. No one would stop you from taking your medicine, nor would they tell you to swap out your pills, so talk about this aspect of your lifestyle early and often.

When people start to catch on, thank them! It's truly the best feeling when people are in your corner and helping. I know that saying thank you may sound silly, but you feel supported when others also advocate for you and you don't feel like the one being an "inconvenience." The first Christmas after Rachael's diagnosis, her parents hosted and cooked gluten-free pasta for the entire family. It was their way of stepping into this new lifestyle with her and showing their support.

We can absolutely assure you that we get messages constantly about this topic.

You don't need to prove anything to anyone, and while the symptoms may not always be obvious or people may just label you as fussy or whatever other adjective they come up with, you are not alone in this. Know that we have a massive community that has your back.

Now, here are some strategies that we have found helpful when eating at gatherings:

- Always offer to bring a dish you know you can eat. This will set you up for success. That way, you know there will always at least be one dish you can rely on.

- Don't go hungry to a gathering. If we didn't have time to prepare a dish before a social gathering, we make sure to eat before we arrive. I can't tell you how many times we've gone to an event where this strategy saved us from disappointment because there wasn't food we could eat, and also from overeating later because we were starving by the time we got home. There's nothing worse than having to socialize with the in-laws while you're hangry.

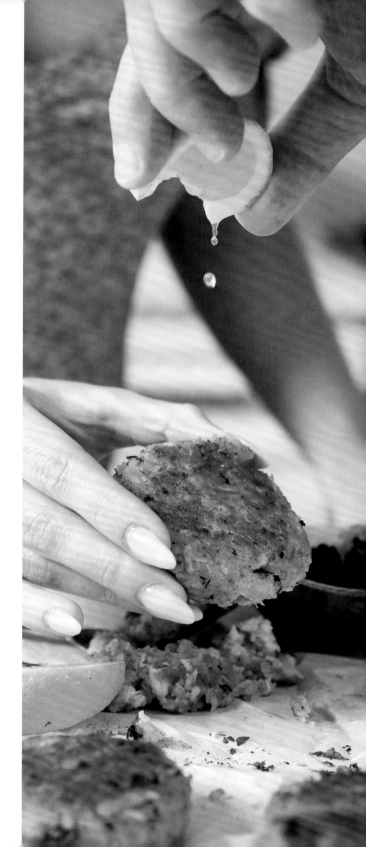

CHAPTER 5

STAPLE TECHNIQUES AND RECIPES

TOM: I often get asked if I am a chef. And the answer is, only in the eyes of Rachael. When I was 23 years old, I moved away from home to start my career. I didn't know anyone within 4 hours of where I was living. I needed a hobby, something to help me relax at the end of the day. There was a co-op grocery store at the corner of the street I lived on, so out of convenience, it was a place where I often stopped in to check out what they had. I started with slow cooker meals. The first meal I remember making was an eight-bean chili—it was terrible. I wasn't exactly off to a good start, but I loved putting on some music, having a glass of wine, and just cooking. It quickly became what I looked forward to each day . . . especially after I met Rachael.

Meeting Rachael was the spark that brought it to the next level. From her vegetarian phase all the way to the PCOS diagnosis, it challenged me as a cook to look at new techniques and, most importantly, learn about food from a different perspective. I did after all brag to her before our first date that I was a "pretty good cook, so she won't have to worry about that." This chapter is hopefully a shortcut through some of the growing pains I experienced, complete with some staple recipes at the end of the chapter.

COOKING TECHNIQUES

How we prepare certain foods during each phase of the menstrual cycle aids in the digestion process and supports healthy hormones. This will be your reference guide to understanding some of the basic cooking techniques you'll find throughout our recipes.

GRILLING

Grilling is a method of cooking food over direct heat. You can use various sources of heat for grilling: wood burning, coals, gas flame, or electric heating. Who doesn't love grill marks?

BAKING

Baking means cooking food items in an oven using dry heat. The dry heat involved in the baking process makes the outside of the food turn brown and keeps the moisture locked in. This method of cooking is used for foods like bread, cakes, cookies, muffins, lasagna, casseroles, and desserts. While technically the same as roasting, baking is at lower temperature.

ROASTING

Roasting, similar to baking, involves the use of an oven at high heat—under 500°F (260°C)—to cook the food, usually meats and vegetables. It quickly becomes browned and dry on the outside, locking most of the moisture inside the food.

BROILING

The broiling element of an oven uses extremely high heat directly above the food. Browning food under the broiler happens quickly, locking in juices and flavor and leaving a crisp exterior. While broiling, keep an eye on the food because it cooks quickly and can burn easily.

SEARING

Typically for meats and fish, this technique browns and caramelizes the outside while leaving the inside uncooked, which helps to lock flavor and moisture inside the protein. Searing happens in a skillet or heavy-bottomed pot over high heat with a cooking fat.

SAUTÉING

I use this technique for almost everything I cook. The food (usually chopped vegetables and aromatics) is cooked in very little oil or fat in a shallow pan over relatively high heat until tender and browned. This method includes tossing and moving the food to achieve even browning. Make sure the oil or fat is hot before adding the food, and don't overcrowd the pan because too much moisture will prevent browning.

FRYING

This means cooking your food in fat. There are several variations of frying:

- Deep-frying, where the food is completely immersed in hot oil until fully cooked and browned on the outside.

- Stir-frying, where you fry the food very quickly over high heat in an oiled pan until cooked or tender-crisp.

- Pan-frying, where food is cooked in a frying pan with a light layer of oil.

- Shallow-frying, where the oil is only about a quarter- to a half-inch deep in the pan. The food is cooked on one side first before being turned over to the other side so it can be completely cooked.

BOILING

Liquid over high heat will begin boiling when the liquid reaches 212°F (100°C). The vigorous bubbling of boiling liquid keeps food moving while it's submerged, giving it a quick, even cook.

SIMMERING

This involves cooking liquid on the stove in a pot or pan usually between 180°F and 205°F (70–96°C). This heat is just below the boiling point and will produce constant small bubbles.

POACHING

This involves cooking food—usually fish, eggs, or fruit—in a hot liquid, usually water, but you can use broth, stock, and juice, too. The liquid needs to be heated between 160°F and 180°F (70–82°C), and the food will remain submerged until completely cooked through.

BLANCHING

Blanching and boiling are almost the same, but in blanching, you remove the food when it is partly cooked through. Usually blanched food is then submerged in an ice bath to stop the cooking process. All sorts of vegetables can be blanched, such as green beans, asparagus, potatoes, and our favorite: brussels sprouts. Blanching helps food keep it's vibrant color, even after it's been cooked, which is lost in some other cooking methods.

STEAMING

This is the process of cooking your food by the steam generated from boiling water. It is handy to have a steamer—a heat-safe strainer (where the food is placed) set above a pot of boiling water with a lid.

BRAISING

Meat is first seared over a high temperature, then cooked in a pan of liquid (water, broth, or stock), covered. The food is cooked at a low temperature for an extended cook time until tender. Roasts and tougher proteins are good for braising.

STEWING

Stewing is when smaller cuts of meat are partially submerged in a liquid at low heat and cooked for a long time. As the stew cooks, fibrous vegetables break down and fat and collagen from the meat melts away. The result is a thick, flavorful gravy filled with tender bites of meat and soft vegetables. It is great for cheaper meats and poultry to add tenderness and flavor for protein that is not suitable for grilling.

DEGLAZING

This is a cooking technique for removing and dissolving browned food residue stuck to the bottom of a pan. The brown bits are released with a small amount of wine, broth, or stock, as you scrape the bottom of the pan with a wooden spoon. Deglazing infuses flavor to sauces, soups, and gravies.

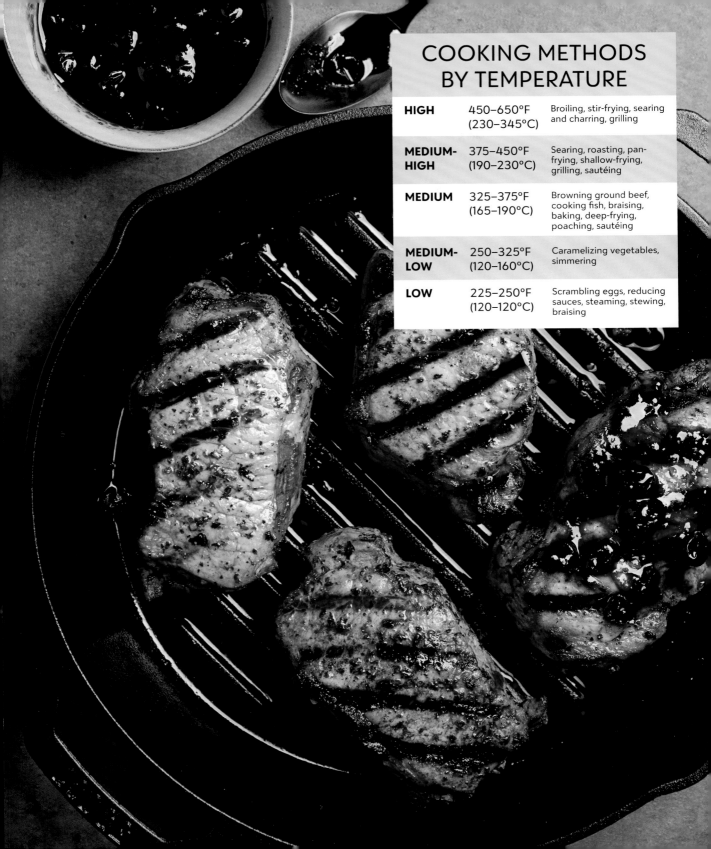

COOKING METHODS BY TEMPERATURE

HIGH	450–650°F (230–345°C)	Broiling, stir-frying, searing and charring, grilling
MEDIUM-HIGH	375–450°F (190–230°C)	Searing, roasting, pan-frying, shallow-frying, grilling, sautéing
MEDIUM	325–375°F (165–190°C)	Browning ground beef, cooking fish, braising, baking, deep-frying, poaching, sautéing
MEDIUM-LOW	250–325°F (120–160°C)	Caramelizing vegetables, simmering
LOW	225–250°F (120–120°C)	Scrambling eggs, reducing sauces, steaming, stewing, braising

FATS BY SMOKE POINT

Refined Avocado   520°F | 270°C

Unrefined Avocado,   480°F | 250°C
Beef Fat

Refined Coconut   450°F | 230°C

Sesame   410°F | 210°C

Extra-Virgin Olive   375°F | 190°C
Chicken Fat, Duck Fat   375°F | 190°C
Lard   370°F | 188°C

Unrefined Coconut   350°F | 175°C

Butter   300°F | 150°C

COOKING FATS BY SMOKE POINT

Have you put much thought into the oils you cook with? Functional nutrition experts will tell you to stay away from highly processed and hydrogenated seed, soybean, canola, corn, sunflower, and vegetable oils. Studies are demonstrating these to be inflammatory and very bad for your heart and vascular system. Because they are highly processed and therefore lacking nutrients, we want to incorporate healthier cooking oils that may offer added health benefits: extra-virgin olive oil, coconut oil, avocado oil, and animal fats.

Not only does the *type* of oil you choose matter, but so does the temperature at which you cook it. Have you ever left oil in a pan on high heat for too long to find it smoking up the kitchen? (Don't worry, every cook will experience setting off the smoke alarm at some point in their journey.) What this means is the oil has reached its smoke point, the temperature at which the oil starts smoking and losing its positive health effects. If you heat oil past its smoke point, you have two problems coming your way. First, say goodbye to the taste and flavor of your dish. We don't compromise taste and flavor in the Sullivan household, and neither should you. Secondly, the nutrients in the oil that are beneficial degrade and the oil will release compounds called free radicals, which are extremely harmful to your body.

PANTRY AND KITCHEN SWAPS

Being healthy is an intentional practice that doesn't happen on accident. It's a habit that has to be formed from consciously choosing to do something repeatedly because it makes you feel good. I want to reiterate this as many times as I can throughout the book because this is not a 30-day fix. This is a lifestyle change and one that requires conscious effort until it becomes a habit. Choosing to set yourself up for success is something we believe in, so we want to help you choose items in your pantry and kitchen that we feel confident will make the swap an easy transition without compromising your tastebuds.

FLOURS

I am going to keep this straightforward because I couldn't be happier that so many brands have *amazing* gluten-free blends. These wheat-flour alternatives are comparable in taste and are made with all real ingredients. I used to try to make my own gluten-free blends, and it was brutal. Almond flour by itself is too grainy. Tapioca or arrowroot starches make for weird textures. Combining them all in a sure-fire way is an endeavor I choose to leave behind.

Our favorite flour substitutes:

We turn to Bob's Red Mill, King Arthur Baking, Pamela's, and Krusteaz. Among these brands you'll have an array of cup-for-cup replacements, as well as baking, pizza, and pancake mixes. For making a roux or slurry to thicken sauces or soups, I prefer arrowroot starch. Whisk a small spoonful with fat, broth, or water, and it should make anything thicker without any lumps.

PASTA

This has to be one of the most commonly asked food swaps we get. First off, let's make it clear that boxed gluten-free pasta has come *so far*. Lots of stores even have gluten-free aisles with several options, and we've done our fair share of sampling. Our most important tip for dried gluten-free pasta: *You can't trust the cook time on the package!* You absolutely must start checking if it's done at least 3 minutes before the recommend cook time. It quickly goes from al dente to broken, mushy pieces. If you have cooked gluten-free pasta, you know what I'm talking about. Also, just like regular pasta, gluten-free pasta is still starchy. Don't rinse it after draining because the starch will help the sauce bind to the pasta.

> *Our favorite pasta substitutes:*
>
> The clear winner based on tasting like the real deal is any Barilla gluten-free product (made from corn and rice), but we also love Jovial (made from brown rice), Ancient Harvest (made from corn, brown rice, and quinoa), and Cappello's (made from almond flour).

SALT

Table salt is very low in trace minerals and can contain unwanted additives. There are amazing pure, mineral-rich, and tasty salts on the market. Like pepper, we like to buy crystal salts and use a grinder to keep the flavor intact.

> *Our favorite salt substitutes:*
>
> When a recipe calls for salt, we use sea or kosher salt. If we want to add extra salt to our plate, we use Himalayan salt.

SUGAR

You'll come across many recipes that call for sugar, so we want to share alternatives that are less processed and more nutritious than refined white sugar and artificial sweeteners.

> *Our favorite sugar substitutes:*
>
> Our favorite sweeteners are coconut sugar, maple syrup, and most of all honey. Each substitute has its place depending on the recipe. A good local honey is the most universal and has the benefit of trace amounts of local pollens, which are good for boosting your immune system against allergens in your area. If you happen to have plant-based allergies, agave syrup is a great substitute you can use. Is it a very low-allergy food that is another good sweetener.

GLUTEN-FREE BREAD, BREADCRUMBS, AND CROUTONS

Admittedly, gluten-free breads can still be fairly overprocessed, and we try to limit our consumption. That being said, eating for PCOS is a lifestyle, and we still want our life to have sandwiches, toasts, and bagels in moderation. We've found storing our breads in the freezer is the best way to prolong freshness. Check out your local grocer to see if the bakery makes their own gluten-free bread.

We use to avoid some of our favorite foods, including meatballs, crabcakes, and chicken fingers, not realizing that simply swapping out the breadcrumbs would make these foods gluten-free. Gluten-free breadcrumbs are one of my pantry necessities.

Our favorite gluten-free bread substitutes:

If you're not interested in making your own gluten-free breads, there are many options on the market. Gluten-free breadcrumbs are widely available. Our favorite brand is Aleia's. Our favorite sourdough bread ships from a bakery called Coco Bakes. If you have access to a Trader Joe's, they have amazing gluten-free bagels. O'Doughs carries a wide line of gluten-free bread products such as bagels, hot dog buns, and loaves that can be found in stores as well as ordered online.

Homemade Croutons

The best way to repurpose the end of a bag of bread is to make croutons. They taste better than any store-bought croutons we've ever had. Rachael has even been known to stick them in her purse to toss on top of restaurant salads. She's a certified classy lady.

4–6 slices of gluten-free bread, cut into ½-in (1.25cm) cubes
¼ cup extra-virgin olive oil
½ tsp dried oregano
½ tsp ground thyme
½ tsp onion powder
½ tsp garlic powder
Salt and pepper, to taste

1 Preheat the oven to 400°F (200°C).

2 Line a baking sheet with parchment paper.

3 Add all of the ingredients to a bowl and gently toss. Spread evenly on the baking sheet.

4 Bake for 15 to 20 minutes, turning halfway through. Enjoy! Leftovers freeze great.

Tip: For breadcrumbs, just throw the croutons in a food processor and pulse a few times.

ICE CREAM

As you have learned by now, Rachael has a sweet tooth. Ice cream is one of those items that we enjoy after dinner every couple of weeks. Luckily, many brands are starting to come out with gluten-free and dairy-free ice creams, but you still have to be on the lookout for the excess sugars and additivities, so double check your labels. Some dairy-free ice creams will contain gluten, and vice versa. There are even some awesome gluten-free ice cream cones on the market. Look for ice cream made with almond milk, cashew milk, coconut milk, avocados, and oat milk. Sorbets (fruit-based) are dairy-free, too. We have made avocado ice cream at home, which is so easy and delicious (but only holds up for a day or two).

Our favorite ice cream substitutes:

Our favorite brands are So Delicious Dairy Free (made with a variety of dairy-free milks), Jeni's dairy-free selections (made with coconut cream), and Cado (made with avocados). Lastly, don't forget your sugar cones! We like Let's Do Gluten Free brand sugar cones.

MILK

Pretty much any grocery store you walk into today has a full section of dairy-free alternatives made with everything from almonds, cashews, and macadamias, to oats, rice, and hemp. Your milk substitute should not contain inflammatory ingredients or sugar that can cause insulin issues. Store-bought dairy-free milks tend to be loaded with sugar, carrageenan, and other preservatives and stabilizers that we want to avoid. However, there are still some great brands with clean ingredients.

Our favorite milk substitutes:

We think almond milk has the best consistency. Always choose unsweetened options. Our favorite brands are Three Trees, MALK, and Elmhurst.

CHEESE

We *use to* have a fully-stocked cheese drawer in the fridge at all times, so cutting out dairy was a big deal for us. I won't lie—we really miss some good cheeses with a charcuterie board, on pizza, or for macaroni and cheese, but we've found some really killer recipes to work around it. (Check out the mac and cheese recipe on our Instagram—it was even allowed at the Thanksgiving table!)

I truly believe cheese has become the new salt, meaning that people use it as a seasoning to mask bland taste—especially in prepared gluten-free foods. There are plenty of ways to achieve the cheesy taste without the dairy. Nutritional yeast, for example, has a great umami, cheesy taste that's both very nutritious (high in B vitamins), as well as a really good cheese-flavor substitute.

Store-bought dairy-free cheese substitutes have gone through more processing than we'd prefer, but they do the trick when you have a craving. However, if we are on a hard reset trying to get Rachael's hormones on track, we steer clear of them.

Most dairy-free cheeses will not melt like standard cheese, so you may have to cook them a bit longer.

Our favorite cheese substitutes:

Sprinkle on some nutritional yeast for a flavor boost.

For store-bought brands, we like Follow Your Heart grated and shredded parmesan. I swear I would think it was the real deal in a side-by-side blind taste test. We use it to top our pizza or pasta. Daiya and 365 by Whole Foods Market are our favorite shredded cheese products. For cheese slices, we turn to Violife. I can't even tell their smoked provolone is vegan. Anything by Miyoko's, from cheese to butter, is tasty. Tofutti's Better Than Ricotta Cheese is our favorite ricotta replacement. Lastly, for queso dips, we prefer cashew-based recipes. Luckily there are tons of simple recipes online that are made with all-natural ingredients that are worth researching. We love Siete Foods cashew-based queso.

YOGURT

Yogurt now comes in a wide variety of options made with coconut, oats, almonds, cashews, and more, all while still providing probiotics to help support a healthy gut. We have spent a lot of time trying all the different store-bought dairy-free yogurts out there, and we've been very happy with both taste and texture across the board. Be mindful of added sugars and when possible, and don't forget you can sweeten them up at home!

Our favorite yogurt substitutes:

When making cold dips, I tend to stick with the nut-based yogurts. When eating it plain with nuts, seeds, and fruits, then go with whatever your palette is feeling. For flavored yogurt, we love Siggis or Lavva. For plain thick yogurt, we like Cocojune. For cooking, we love to use Forager because the runny texture makes for great sauces and dips. When we are cooking sauces over heat that we want to thicken, I use coconut milk.

BUTTER

Butter contains dairy, too, so don't forget to sub it out! As someone who cooks, this replacement may have been even harder than cheese because butter is used in damn near everything.

Ghee or clarified butter is made from regular cow's butter, which has been melted at a low heat so the milk solids separate and can be strained out. You can purchase this at the store or make it at home. Here is the dilemma: it tastes and works great and is very low in dairy and is even touted as anti-inflammatory, but it's not completely dairy-free—some low levels of lactose and casein remain. You might find you have absolutely no reaction to it, so I would experiment and see if it's problematic. There isn't great research on this, so in the meantime, we use ghee sparingly.

Our favorite butter substitutes:

For store-bought butter replacements, there are several vegan options we turn to. Miyoko's brand is a clear winner in our hearts. Earth Balance is another excellent option. We have noticed that many vegan and plant-based butters contain soy, so we always read our labels and avoid that.

MAYONNAISE

I've been told that making homemade mayonnaise is life changing, but so far I'm holding out on that life change and keeping it in my back pocket for a rainy day. For the ultimate control of your mayo though—make your own! It's essentially just an emulsion of egg yolk, oil, and acid. If you're going to buy store-bought like we do, look for real ingredients. Many of the of the big brand names use oils that are not what we would like to see. Soybean oil is the biggest culprit. Make sure you check your labels because sometimes it will say olive or avocado oil on the front, but the ingredients list shows it's still been cut with soybean oil.

Our favorite mayo substitutes:

There are lots of high-quality mayos at the store, but our favorites are Primal Kitchen and Sir Kensington.

SOY SAUCE

It is one of those controversial ingredients because the more you search, the more you can find acclaimed positive and negative benefits. It seems like every other week there are new articles talking about the dangers of soy, specifically dealing with estrogen levels. The long and short from our view is that there are substitutes that aren't so widely debated like coconut aminos, so we opt for that and avoid soy sauce. Remember, soy sauce or other soy products are also commonly used in processed foods, vegan meats, and dairy-free products, so be on the lookout for these culprits.

Our favorite soy sauce substitute:

We love coconut aminos. Our favorite brand is Bragg Coconut Liquid Aminos.

KETCHUP AND BARBECUE SAUCE

Ketchup and barbecue sauce aren't the healthiest condiments on the block, but that doesn't mean you have to say goodbye to delicious BBQ brisket, ribs, and chicken. Look for unsweetened brands or brands with the lowest amount of added sugar.

Our favorite condiment substitutes:

For ketchup, you can make your own or look for brands that have little to no sugar and added flavors. We enjoy Primal Kitchen, Sir Kensington, and Annie's.

For barbecue sauce, we almost always choose to make our own. We even have a recipe for you. Our favorite type is mustard or vinegar based. Some brands that offer little or no sugar options are Simple Truth, Primal Kitchen, Good Food For Good, G Hughes, and Lillie's Q. Many larger brands are also opting in to sugar-free, so check out those labels.

Barbecue Sauce

Barbecue sauce is typically loaded with sodium and sugar. It's a big reason why eating barbecue gets a bad wrap. On the flip side, it is easy to make clean versions that taste amazing! This one with a mustard/vinegar base is my favorite.

1 cup yellow mustard
½ cup honey
½ cup apple cider vinegar
¼ cup ketchup
1 tsp garlic powder
½ tsp salt
Dash of hot sauce

1 In a medium saucepan, whisk together all ingredients.

2 Bring together over low heat for 3 to 5 minutes.

3 Allow it to cool, and store in a jar in the refrigerator for up to 2 weeks.

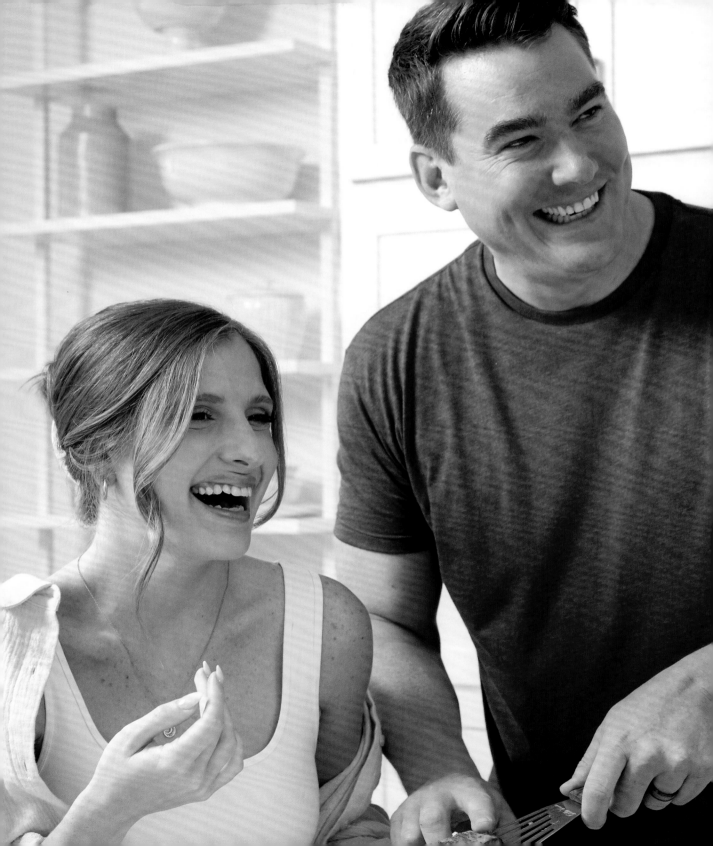

SALAD DRESSING 4 WAYS

MAKES: about ¾ cup
PREP TIME: 5 minutes
COOK TIME: none

Simple vinaigrette base:
½ cup extra-virgin olive oil
¼ cup vinegar (red, balsamic, white, or apple cider)
½ tsp sea salt
½ tsp freshly cracked black pepper

Rachael bought me a salad dressing mixer as a stocking stuffer for Christmas one year, and I never realized how easy making homemade dressings could be. Warning: this is an addiction. Here are four simple salad dressings, and each one uses the simple vinaigrette base.

1 For each of the options, whisk or shake together thoroughly before using.

2 Store in an airtight container for 1 to 2 weeks. Remove from the fridge 5 minutes before using, then shake to reincorporate.

Apple cider vinaigrette dressing:
Simple vinaigrette base (using apple cider vinegar)
1 tbsp Dijon mustard
2 tbsp honey
1 garlic clove, minced

Balsamic vinaigrette:
Simple vinaigrette base (using balsamic vinegar)
1 tbsp Dijon mustard
2 tbsp honey
1 garlic clove, minced

Red wine vinaigrette:
Simple vinaigrette base (using red wine vinegar)
1 tsp Dijon mustard
1 garlic clove, minced
½ tbsp honey
1 tsp dried oregano

White wine vinaigrette:
Simple vinaigrette base (using white wine vinegar)
1 tsp Dijon mustard
1 tsp honey
1 shallot, minced

Tip: These salad dressings will separate when put in the refrigerator. We suggest using canning jars or dressing mixers so you can easily shake and mix back up.

YOGURT BOWLS

SERVES: 1
PREP TIME: 5 minutes
COOK TIME: none

Yogurt bowls are Rachael's favorite way to start the day and align with her cycle. Each bowl consists of different combinations tailored to specific phases. Have fun creating your morning bowls, and don't be afraid to mix it up. Play with seasonal fruits and toppings depending on the phase you're in. The following combos are her favorite for each phase.

Start with your bowl of dairy-free yogurt. Stir in or arrange the various ingredients on top as desired, and enjoy.

Menstrual:
Bowl of dairy-free yogurt
Flaxseeds
Pumpkin seeds
Blueberries or blackberries
Cacao nibs

Follicular:
Bowl of dairy-free yogurt
Flaxseeds
Pumpkin seeds
Crushed cashews
Cashew butter
Pomegranate seeds

Ovulatory:
Bowl of dairy-free yogurt
Sesame seeds
Sunflower seeds
Shredded coconut
Slivered almonds and/or
  pecan halves
Almond butter
Raspberries or strawberries

Luteal:
Bowl of dairy-free yogurt
Sesame seeds
Sunflower seeds
Walnuts
Honey
Bananas or peaches

SHEET PAN 4 WAYS

SERVES: 2
PREP TIME: 10 minutes
COOK TIME: 15–30 minutes

Every time I had to go on a work trip for a couple of days and Rachael was home alone to fend for herself, there was one thing I could absolutely count on: Rachael would make a sheet pan meal. It takes under 10 minutes to prep, requires minimal effort, and won't leave your sink full of dishes. These are also great meal prep ideas. In honor of Rachael's favorite go-to meal, here is a quick recipe for each phase. We love topping each of these sheet pan recipes with Rachael's Tahini Dressing.

Rachael's Tahini Dressing:
In a small bowl, whisk together ⅓ cup tahini, juice of 1 medium lemon (or about 3 tablespoons), and salt and pepper to taste. Slowly add 3 to 5 tablespoons lukewarm water, whisking until creamy and pourable.

Menstrual:
1 bunch kale, ribs discarded, torn
1 tbsp olive oil
8 oz (225g) sliced baby bella mushrooms
1 (15oz/425g) can chickpeas, drained and rinsed
1 garlic clove, minced
1 tsp dried thyme
Salt and freshly cracked black pepper, to taste
Rice (optional), to serve

1 Preheat the oven to 350°F (180°C). Line a baking sheet with parchment paper.

2 Place the kale on the baking sheet. Drizzle the olive oil over, toss to coat, and massage with your hands to soften the kale. Add the remaining ingredients, and toss to coat.

3 Cook for 10 to 15 minutes, tossing halfway through. Rachael prefers it crispy, so we broil it for about 2 minutes, watching the food carefully so it doesn't burn.

4 Add to a bowl over rice (if desired). Drizzle with Rachael's Tahini Dressing, and enjoy.

Follicular:

1 sweet potato, diced

1 tbsp olive oil, divided

Salt and freshly cracked black pepper, to taste

6 oz (170g) chicken breast

Juice from 1 lemon

1½ tsp Italian seasoning, divided

1 tsp garlic powder

2 cups broccoli florets

Rice (optional), to serve

1 Preheat the oven to 425°F (220°C). Line a baking sheet with parchment paper.

2 Place the sweet potatoes on the sheet. Drizzle with ½ tablespoon olive oil, and season with salt and pepper. Toss to coat evenly. Roast for 12 minutes.

3 Meanwhile, season the chicken with the lemon juice, ¾ teaspoon of the Italian seasoning, and the garlic powder.

4 In a medium bowl, toss the broccoli with the remaining olive oil. Toss in the remaining Italian seasoning.

5 Remove the sweet potatoes from the oven and add the chicken and broccoli to the same sheet. Roast for an additional 15 minutes or until the chicken is cooked through. Rachael prefers it crispy, so we broil it for about 2 minutes, watching carefully so it doesn't burn.

6 Add to a bowl over rice (if desired). Drizzle with Rachael's Tahini Dressing, and enjoy.

Ovulatory:

6 oz (170g) chicken breast, cut into 1-in (2.5cm) slices

1½ tsp olive oil, divided

1 tsp Italian seasoning

8 oz (225g) brussels sprouts, stems removed, sliced vertically into ¼-in (0.5cm) slices

6–8 asparagus spears, ends removed, cut into 1-in (2.5cm) pieces

1 tbsp balsamic vinegar

1 garlic clove, minced

Salt and freshly cracked black pepper, to taste

Rice (optional), to serve

1 Preheat the oven to 425°F (220°C). Line a baking sheet with parchment paper.

2 Add the chicken slices to the middle of the baking sheet. Drizzle with ¾ teaspoon of the olive oil and the Italian seasoning. Toss to coat.

3 In a medium bowl, toss the brussels sprouts and asparagus with the balsamic vinegar, remaining olive oil, garlic, salt, and pepper. Add to the baking sheet around the chicken.

4 Roast for 15 minutes or until the chicken is cooked through.

5 Drizzle with Rachael's Tahini Dressing, and enjoy.

Luteal:

2 cups cauliflower florets

1 cup cooked chickpeas, drained and rinsed

1½ tsp olive oil

Salt and freshly cracked black pepper, to taste

1 tbsp sriracha

½ tsp sesame seeds

Arugula or wild rice (optional), to serve

Chopped green onions (optional), for garnish

1 Preheat the oven to 425°F (220°C). Line a baking sheet with parchment paper.

2 Place the cauliflower and chickpeas on the sheet. Drizzle with the olive oil, salt, pepper, and sriracha. Toss to coat.

3 Roast for 10 minutes. Remove and sprinkle with the sesame seeds. Return to the oven to bake for 3 minutes.

4 Serve over arugula or rice, if desired, and garnish with green onions, if desired. Drizzle with Rachael's Tahini Dressing, and enjoy.

CHAPTER 6

FOODS FOR YOUR MENSTRUAL PHASE

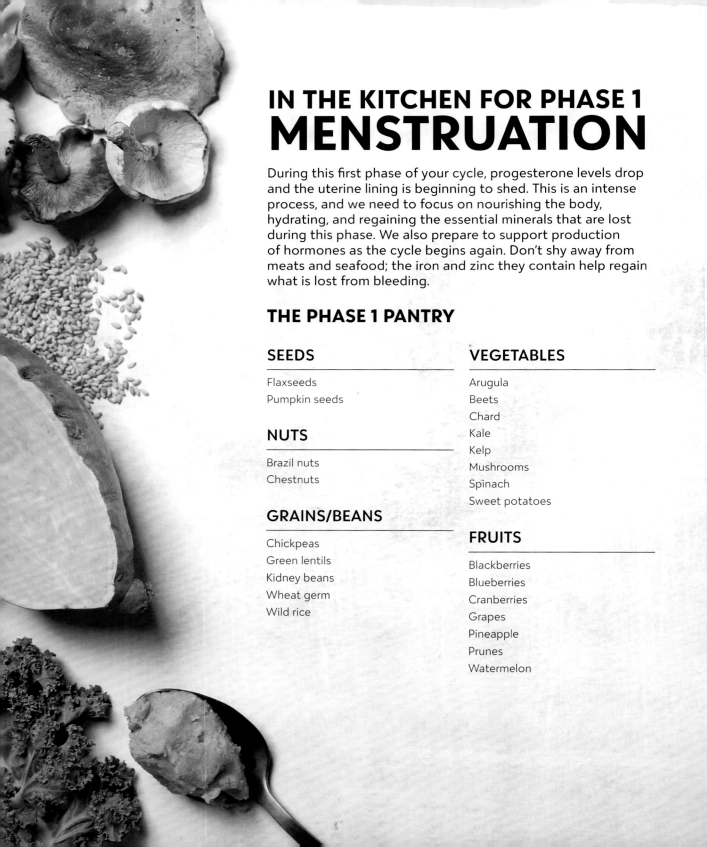

IN THE KITCHEN FOR PHASE 1
MENSTRUATION

During this first phase of your cycle, progesterone levels drop and the uterine lining is beginning to shed. This is an intense process, and we need to focus on nourishing the body, hydrating, and regaining the essential minerals that are lost during this phase. We also prepare to support production of hormones as the cycle begins again. Don't shy away from meats and seafood; the iron and zinc they contain help regain what is lost from bleeding.

THE PHASE 1 PANTRY

SEEDS

Flaxseeds
Pumpkin seeds

NUTS

Brazil nuts
Chestnuts

GRAINS/BEANS

Chickpeas
Green lentils
Kidney beans
Wheat germ
Wild rice

VEGETABLES

Arugula
Beets
Chard
Kale
Kelp
Mushrooms
Spinach
Sweet potatoes

FRUITS

Blackberries
Blueberries
Cranberries
Grapes
Pineapple
Prunes
Watermelon

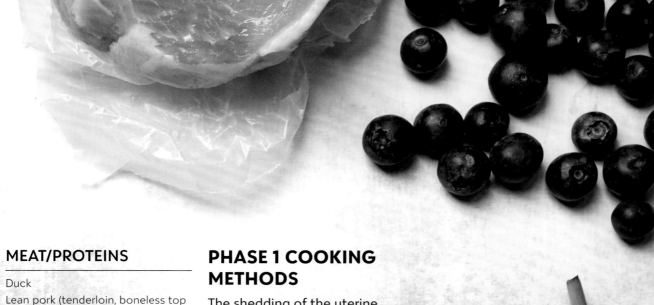

MEAT/PROTEINS

Duck

Lean pork (tenderloin, boneless top loin, or sirloin roast)

Tofu

SEAFOOD

Clams

Crab

Lobster

Mussels

Octopus

Oysters

Salmon

Scallops

OTHER:

Bone broth

Dark chocolate

Light teas (nettle, raspberry leaf, chamomile, and ginger)

Miso

Probiotic yogurts (dairy-free)

Salt

Turmeric

PHASE 1 COOKING METHODS

The shedding of the uterine lining is a very energy-draining process, so we want to give your digestive system a break. You may notice a craving for warmer foods during this time—lean into that! Cold and raw foods tend to be harder to digest. Eat lightly cooked, easy-to-digest foods: gluten-free oatmeal, soups, and stews. Also go for green juices and smoothies that are full of nutrients but easy for your stomach to absorb and digest since they're already partially broken down.

MISO SOUP

SERVES: 2
PREP TIME: 10 minutes
COOK TIME: 25 minutes

4 cups dashi or vegetable broth

5 shiitake mushrooms, stems
  removed, sliced

¼ cup white miso

2 tsp coconut aminos

1 cup roughly chopped kale

5 oz (140g) medium-diced firm tofu

2 green onions, sliced, for garnish

This was the first post on the @Mealssheeats Instagram page and the first time I ever used a hashtag. I had just begun tracking our recipes at this point and becoming consistent with our cooking techniques and styles. Little did we know this meal would be a stepping stone that would launch us into a cookbook and also inform the world that Rachael was in "shark week" (i.e., on her period). Enjoy this miso soup made with simple ingredients that provide an abundance of flavor.

1 In a medium saucepan, bring the broth to a boil. Add the mushrooms, reduce the heat to medium-low, and simmer for 5 minutes.

2 In a small bowl, stir together the miso and coconut aminos until smooth. Stir into the broth, and add the kale and tofu. Cook 1 to 2 minutes longer, being careful not to boil.

3 Pour into serving bowls and garnish with green onions. Serve immediately.

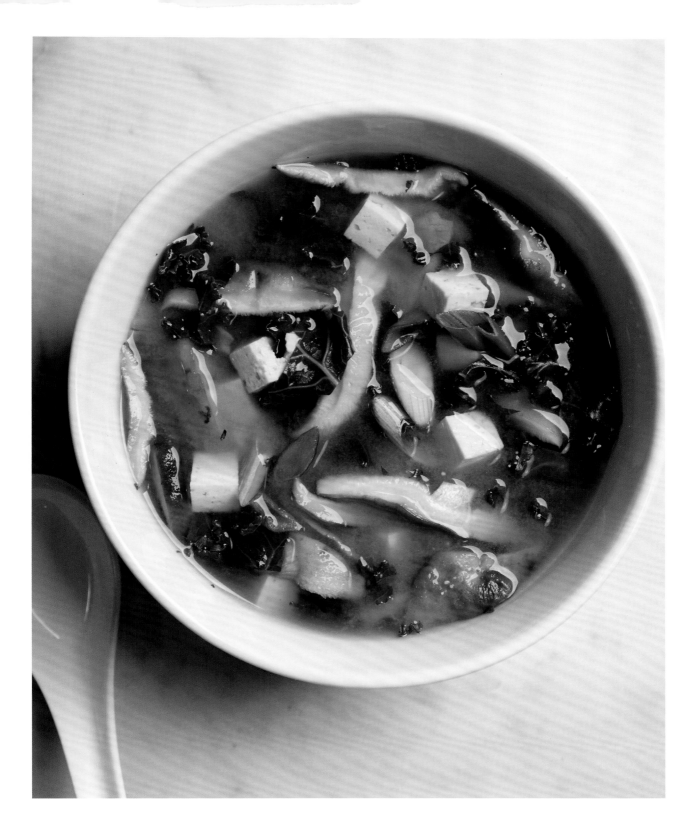

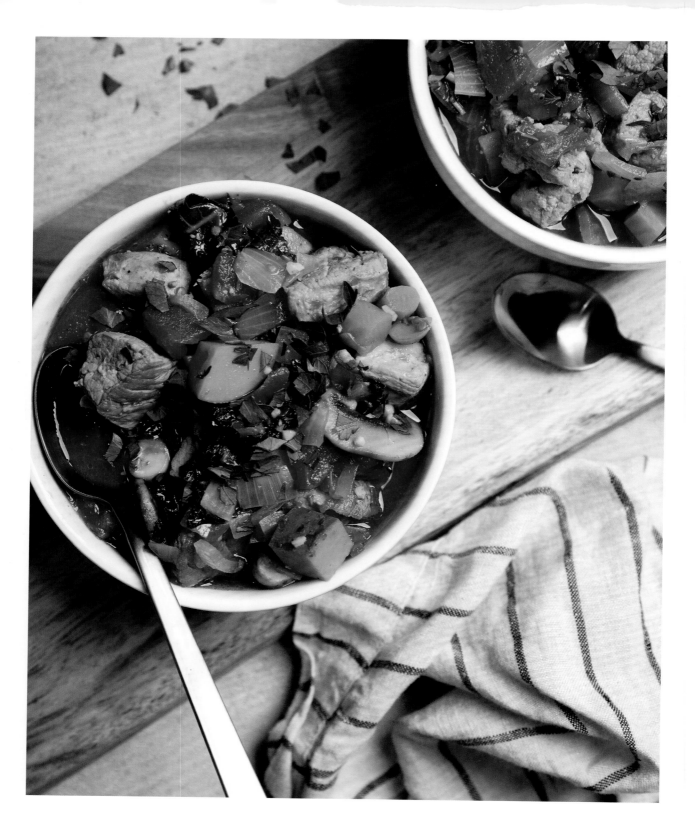

PORK STEW

SERVES: 3–4
PREP TIME: 15 minutes
COOK TIME: 1 hour 20 minutes

1 tbsp extra-virgin olive oil

1 lb (450g) pork top loin or pork tenderloin, cubed

Salt and pepper, to taste

1 small onion, chopped

4 cups chicken broth

1 (14 oz/400g) can diced tomatoes

1 tsp dried rosemary

1 tsp dried oregano

2 garlic cloves, minced

1 bay leaf

½ tsp smoked paprika

1 sweet potato, diced

2 carrots, diced

1 cup shredded kale

1 cup sliced mushrooms (pick your favorite type)

Parsley, to garnish

Stews are just the best! They are easy to get creative with and a way to clear out the refrigerator, not to mention they freeze and reheat well. Obviously, we tend to have stews more in the winter and fall, but when there are a couple stormy days during the spring or summer, it's time to light some candles, throw on a movie, and enjoy a bowl. This stew is a great way to see how flavors can highlight each other. The proteins are seared to get great bold flavors into your pot, but we finish by simmering to cook through. This helps break them down and make them easier for the body to digest. There are mixed opinions on meat during menstruation (high in nutrients but intensive to digest), so we like to stick with leaner cuts during menstruation. This stew is a perfect way to keep your protein high, get your iron in, and make it so the body is not working on overdrive to absorb and digest.

1 In a large Dutch oven or pot, heat the olive oil over medium-high heat. Season the pork with salt and pepper. Working in batches so you don't overcrowd the pan, brown the pork and onion, about 10 minutes.

2 In the pot, stir together the broth, tomatoes, rosemary, oregano, garlic, bay leaf, paprika, and additional salt and pepper to taste, along with the pork and onions. Deglaze the pan. Allow the stew to come to a boil, then reduce the heat to medium-low or where the stew is at a simmer. Cover and let simmer for 40 minutes.

3 Add the sweet potato, carrots, kale, and mushrooms to the pot. Increase heat to medium-high, bring the stew to a boil, then reduce the heat to medium-low and simmer for 30 minutes or until the vegetables are tender.

4 Thicken if desired (see the note), and serve hot, garnished with parsley.

NOTE

To thicken your stew, make a slurry of 1 tablespoon cornstarch and 1 tablespoon water, and thoroughly stir into the stew at the end of the cooking time. You can add more, but note that the stew will naturally, slowly thicken over time.

BEET SALAD

SERVES: 3–4
PREP TIME: 35 minutes
COOK TIME: 50 minutes

3–4 medium-large red or golden beets (uncooked)

4 tbsp extra-virgin olive oil, divided

⅓ cup very finely chopped red onion

1 garlic clove, finely minced

2 tbsp red wine vinegar or apple cider vinegar

1 navel orange (2 tbsp zest and 4 tbsp juice), plus more zest for garnish

½ cup raisins or dried cranberries

1 cup chopped mint leaves, plus more for garnish

½ tsp salt, plus more to taste

½ tsp pepper, plus more to taste

1 cup shelled and gently crushed pistachios

TOM: Let's take a moment to talk about feeling tired and run down during the menstrual phase. There used to be days when Rachael literally could not get out of bed. I was so torn about how to help her. Does she want me encourage her to toughen up and push through? Do I bring the heating pad and rub her back? It's a brutal situation, and as a husband, I had zero guidance on how to support Rachael. I know now that the body is working extra hard during this phase of the cycle, and resources are being depleted, but add on top of that a hormone imbalance due to PCOS, and it's an extra-trying situation. This beet salad, both refreshing and delicious, is nutrient dense and easy for your body to process and absorb during this depleting phase. This can also be made a day ahead and enjoyed cold.

1 Preheat the oven to 425°F (220°C). Cut the leafy tops off the beets, leaving ½ inch (1.25cm) of the stem on. Wash the beets well.

2 Toss the beets in 1 tablespoon olive oil, and season with salt and pepper if desired. Individually wrap each beet tightly in foil. Place the wrapped beets on a baking sheet, and roast until fork-tender, 40 to 50 minutes.

3 Remove from the oven and carefully open the foil (be cautious of steam). Allow to cool for 5 minutes. Peel while still warm, using a paper towel to grab the skin. Chop into wedges or ½-inch (1.25cm) cubes. Place in a large serving bowl.

4 To the same large bowl, add the red onion, garlic, remaining 3 tablespoons olive oil, vinegar, orange zest and orange juice, raisins, mint, and the ½ teaspoon each of salt and pepper. Toss to combine well. Mix in the pistachios.

5 Taste and add more of any ingredients. Garnish with some additional fresh mint and orange zest. Serve and enjoy.

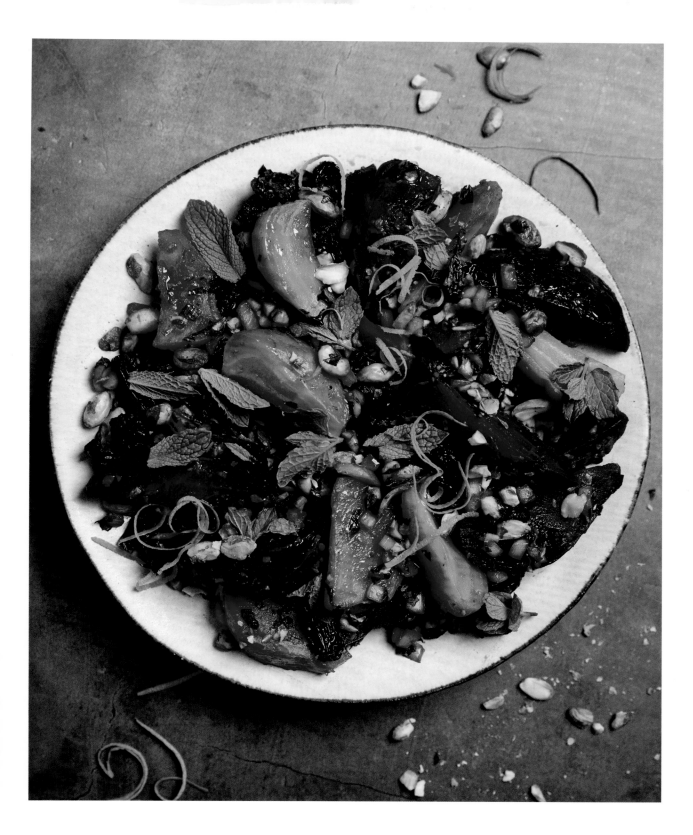

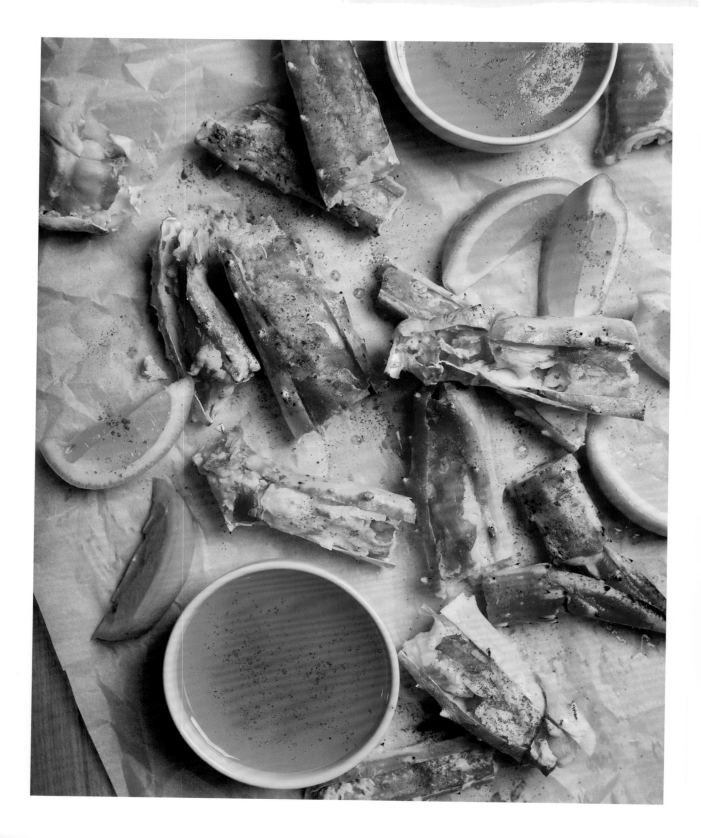

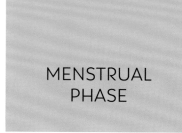

BAKED KING CRAB LEGS
WITH "BUTTER" SAUCE

SERVES: 2 or 4 for an appetizer
PREP TIME: 10 minutes
COOK TIME: 20 minutes

2–4 king crab legs (cooked)

1 lemon, sliced into 4 wedges

½ cup dairy-free butter, such as Mykonos

Splash of hot sauce (optional)

1 tsp honey

Smoked paprika, for garnish

RACHAEL: At 6 years old, I was introduced to king crab legs at Heston Supper Club, a staple eatery in the Midwest where my family would stop on our way home from cutting down Christmas trees in Indiana. By age 10, snow crab and king crab were the only birthday meals I ever requested. I even lived through the golden era of Red Lobster's endless snow crab legs for $22.99. My sister Beth and I partook in the franchise's $3 million loss in profits in one year as we would sit for not two helpings, but three or four. After Tom heard that story, suddenly we were eating crab legs on a monthly basis.

1 Preheat the oven to 400°F (200°C). Using kitchen shears, carefully cut the crab legs into 3- to 4-inch (8–10cm) pieces. Cut them again lengthwise to expose the crabmeat.

2 Place the pieces on a baking sheet with the meaty side up. Place 2 lemon wedges on the baking sheet, and loosely cover the sheet with foil to avoid drying out the crab. Bake for 20 minutes.

3 Meanwhile, in a small saucepan, melt the butter over medium-low heat. Stir in the juice from the remaining 2 lemon wedges, along with the honey and the hot sauce (if using).

4 Remove the crab legs from the oven. Squeeze the warmed lemon wedges all over the exposed crab meat. Garnish with smoked paprika. Serve with warm butter sauce.

NOTE
Make the butter sauce up to 1 day in advance. Keep refrigerated, and gently warm when ready to use.

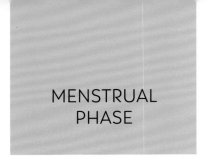

BALSAMIC PORK
WITH BLUEBERRY SAUCE

SERVES: 4
PREP TIME: 40 minutes, plus 1 hour or overnight to marinate
COOK TIME: 15 minutes

1 pork tenderoin
1 tbsp extra-virgin olive oil

Marinade:
⅓ cup balsamic vinegar
2 tbsp water
1 tsp minced garlic
½ tsp salt
½ tsp pepper
⅓ cup extra-virgin olive oil
1½ tsp dried basil
½ tsp dried oregano

Blueberry Sauce:
1 pint fresh or frozen blueberries
¾ cup water
¼ cup honey or maple syrup
Salt, to taste

TOM: Pork has a tendency to be less expensive but it's also kind of boring. This recipe shows off how versatile pork can be. It was one of the first dishes I posted online that I was proud of how it looked, and more importantly how good it tasted. It's great to serve over a bed of arugula or wild rice. Other tasty side dishes include roasted garlic mushrooms, beet salad, and lentil soup.

1 Add all of the marinade ingredients to a large resealable bag.Seal and shake until thoroughly mixed. Add the pork tenderloin, seal the bag, and chill in the refrigerator for at least 1 hour or overnight.

2 When ready to cook the pork tenderloin, remove it from the fridge and let it come to room temperature while you prepare the blueberry sauce. In a small saucepan, combine all of the ingredients. Bring to a boil over medium-high heat, and then reduce to a simmer. Continue to cook until three-fourths of the liquid cooks off, about 10 minutes, stirring periodically. Thin with more water as needed.

3 Preheat oven to 350°F (180°C). Preheat a large cast-iron skillet over medium-high heat. Add the olive oil to the skillet and heat until shimmering. Remove the pork tenderloin from the marinade and add the pork to the pan. Sear for 3 to 4 minutes per side. Resist the urge to move it. Once golden brown, it will release without sticking.

4 Once all sides of the pork are seared, move the skillet to the oven. Bake pork for 25 minutes or until it reaches an internal temperature of 140°F (60°C). Remove pork from the oven and let rest for 10 minutes as the temperature rises to 145°F (63°C).

5 After resting, top with the blueberry sauce and enjoy.

NOTE
You can also grill or bake the tenderloin. To bake, place in an oven preheated to 425°F (220°C) and cook for 10 minutes per side.

You can also use pork chops, but be sure to adjust the cooking time as necessary.

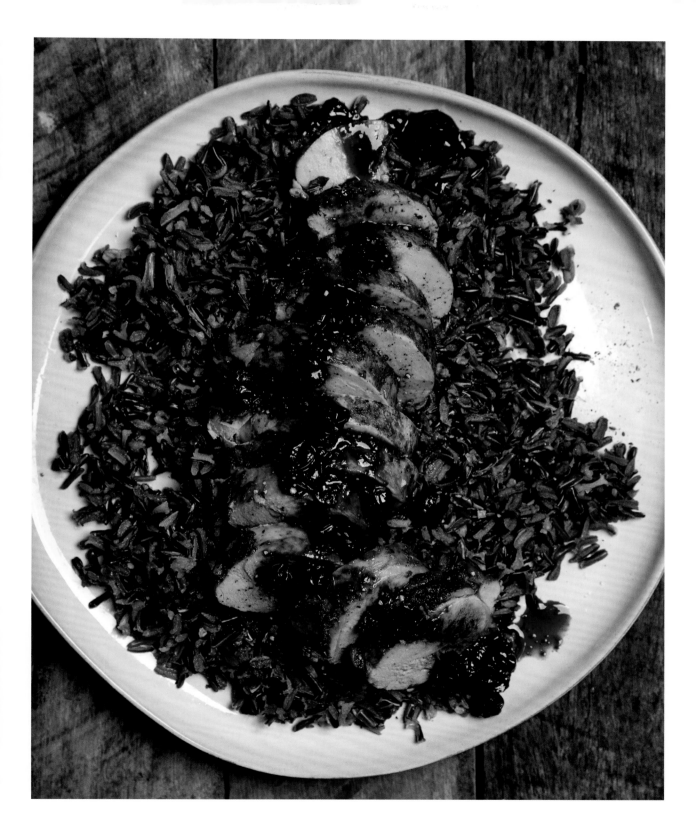

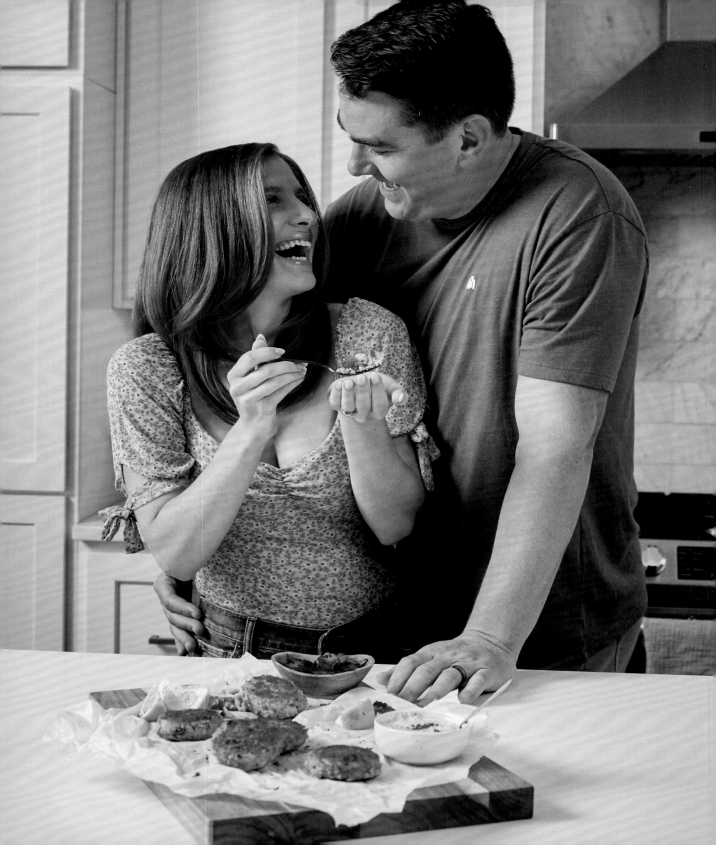

CRAB CAKES
WITH RÉMOULADE

MAKES: 6–8 larger (for dinner) or
15–20 smaller (for appetizer)
PREP TIME: 45 minutes
COOK TIME: 25 minutes

Crab Cakes:

⅓ cup mayonnaise

1 large egg, beaten

1 tsp Dijon mustard

½ tsp Worcestershire sauce

Dash of hot sauce (optional)

½ tbsp Old Bay Seasoning

Salt and pepper, to taste

1 lb (450g) fresh crabmeat

¾ cup gluten-free panko

2 tbsp chopped flat-leaf parsley

1 tbsp dairy-free butter, plus more
  if needed

½ tbsp olive oil, plus more if needed

Rémoulade:

⅔ cup mayonnaise

1 tbsp Dijon mustard

Zest and juice of ½ lemon

2 sweet gherkins, finely diced

1 tbsp diced chives

1 tsp Worcestershire sauce

1 tsp smoked paprika

Salt and pepper, to taste

RACHAEL: For our first wedding anniversary, we celebrated with a weekend getaway to Rhode Island where we stayed in downtown Newport at a bed and breakfast, just within walking distance of the city center. I had my first oyster shooter, my first lobster roll, and indulged in an insane amount of crab cakes here. Just writing about it makes me miss it. The air was a little crisper, the seafood tasted a little fresher, and I loved all the new experiences this place had to offer. Coming home from that trip, we quickly became infatuated with the upper East Coast. The following fall when it was time to celebrate our anniversary, the only place we wanted to explore was a new coastal town. It became our first married tradition. During the months spent at home until we can get a taste of that upper East Coast again, making crab cakes is one of the ways we are able to relive those memories—even if for just a few bites.

1 In a small bowl, whisk together all of the ingredients for the rémoulade. Cover and refrigerate until ready to serve.

2 Prepare the crab cakes. In a medium bowl, whisk together the mayonnaise, egg, mustard, Worcestershire sauce, hot sauce (if using), and Old Bay Seasoning. Season with salt and pepper to taste.

3 To that same bowl, fold in the crabmeat, panko, and parsley. With an ice cream or cookie scoop, form the mixture into balls. A smaller scoop can yield 15 to 20 cakes, and a larger scoop can yield 6 to 8. Flatten slightly to form each scoop into a patty. Place on a plate and refrigerate for at least 30 minutes.

4 In a large skillet over medium-high heat, heat the butter and oil until melted and hot. Working in batches, add the crab cakes, and cook until golden brown and crispy, 4 to 6 minutes per side. Add more butter and olive oil between batches as needed. Serve hot with the rémoulade.

CHAPTER 7

FOODS FOR YOUR FOLLICULAR PHASE

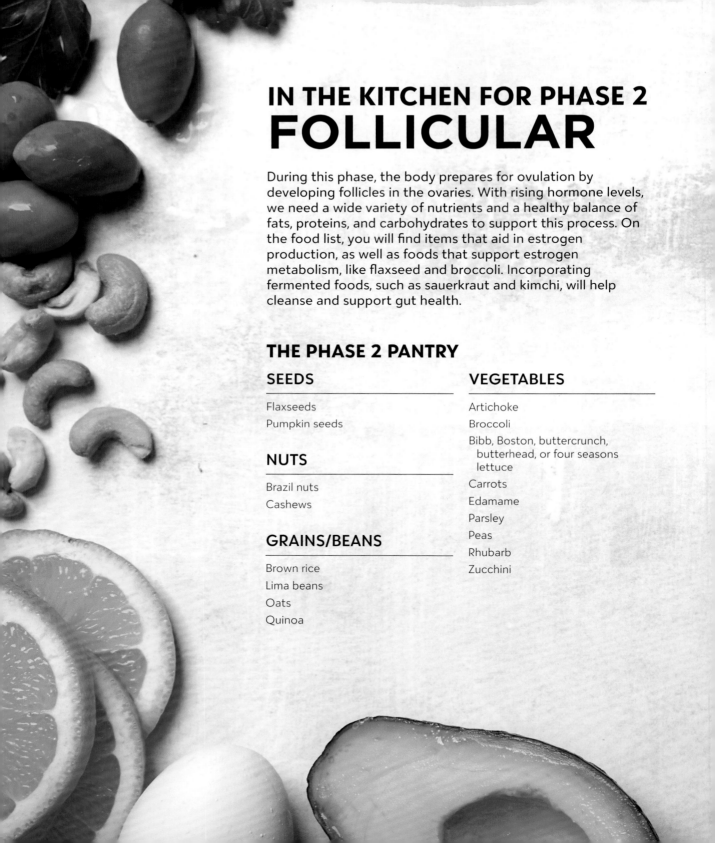

IN THE KITCHEN FOR PHASE 2
FOLLICULAR

During this phase, the body prepares for ovulation by developing follicles in the ovaries. With rising hormone levels, we need a wide variety of nutrients and a healthy balance of fats, proteins, and carbohydrates to support this process. On the food list, you will find items that aid in estrogen production, as well as foods that support estrogen metabolism, like flaxseed and broccoli. Incorporating fermented foods, such as sauerkraut and kimchi, will help cleanse and support gut health.

THE PHASE 2 PANTRY

SEEDS

Flaxseeds
Pumpkin seeds

NUTS

Brazil nuts
Cashews

GRAINS/BEANS

Brown rice
Lima beans
Oats
Quinoa

VEGETABLES

Artichoke
Broccoli
Bibb, Boston, buttercrunch, butterhead, or four seasons lettuce
Carrots
Edamame
Parsley
Peas
Rhubarb
Zucchini

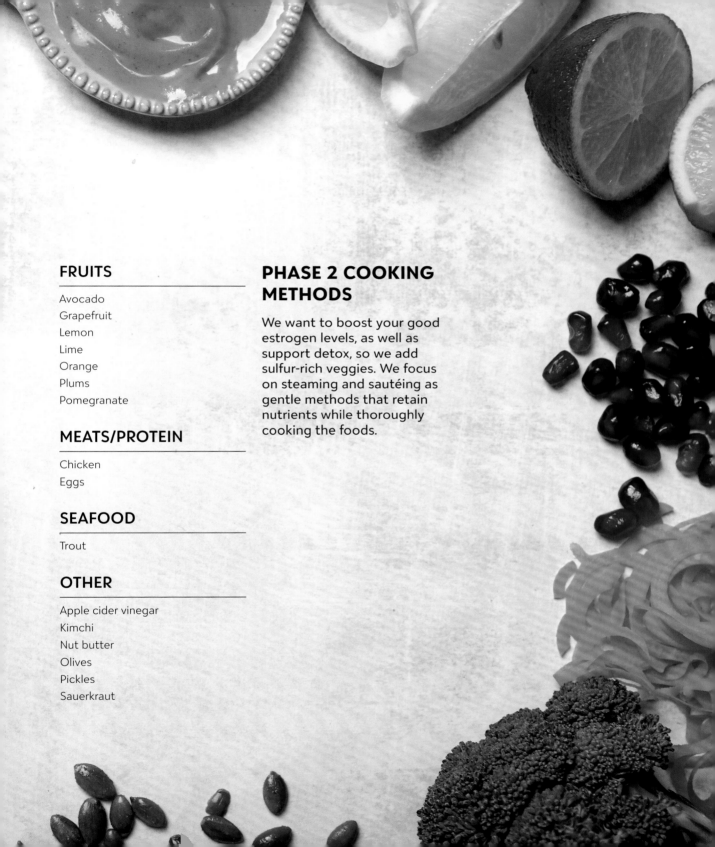

FRUITS

Avocado
Grapefruit
Lemon
Lime
Orange
Plums
Pomegranate

MEATS/PROTEIN

Chicken
Eggs

SEAFOOD

Trout

OTHER

Apple cider vinegar
Kimchi
Nut butter
Olives
Pickles
Sauerkraut

PHASE 2 COOKING METHODS

We want to boost your good estrogen levels, as well as support detox, so we add sulfur-rich veggies. We focus on steaming and sautéing as gentle methods that retain nutrients while thoroughly cooking the foods.

RACHAEL'S PASTA

SERVES: 3–4
PREP TIME: 5 minutes
COOK TIME: 20 minutes

½ box (6 oz/170g) gluten-free spaghetti or angel hair pasta (the thinner the better)

1–2 tbsp extra-virgin olive oil

3 cloves garlic, minced

1 (8 oz/225g) jar julienne-cut sun-dried tomatoes in olive oil with Italian herbs

2 cups finely chopped broccoli florets

1 cup frozen peas

Salt and pepper, to taste

Flat-leaf parsley, finely chopped, to garnish

RACHAEL: Food was a family bonding experience for me growing up, and there was no greater time spent in the kitchen than with my dad making his favorite cuisine: Italian. From his famous vodka sauce to veal parmigiana, he was always cooking Italian-inspired dishes. Although he will tell you my mom's gravy recipe takes the cake, my favorite dish comes down to the simplistic notion of mixing angel hair pasta with a quality olive oil, fresh herbs, and loads of sun-dried tomatoes. The only thing better than my dad's pasta is his day-old pasta after the flavors have marinated together. Please note that you will wake up craving reheated leftovers for breakfast, and if you choose to store your leftovers in a plastic container, the aftermath of olive oil and tomato stains means you made it just right.

1 In a large pot, cook the pasta in boiling salted water until al dente. Drain and reserve 1 cup cooking water.

2 In a medium pan over medium-high heat, add the olive oil and garlic. Cook until fragrant, 30 seconds to 1 minute. Add the sun-dried tomatoes and ½ the oil from the jar. Cook for 1 minute, and then reduce the heat to medium. Add the broccoli and peas, and toss for 1 minute. Cover the pan and let cook for 3 minutes.

3 Add the drained pasta to the pan, and toss to mix over medium heat for 2 to 3 minutes. Add half of the reserved cooking water and simmer for 2 to 4 minutes, stirring occasionally until pasta and sauce are well combined. Season with salt and pepper to taste. Remove the pan from the heat and top with parsley. Serve immediately.

NOTE

My dad, Ed, taught us a twist that elevates this dish and makes it a true comfort meal: pan-frying the pasta! Before adding the pasta to the sauce mixture, in a separate small pan over medium-high heat, add 2 tablespoons olive oil with a spoonful of the sauce mixture and a spoonful of the reserved cooking water. Once hot, drop the pasta in and give it a 2-minute shallow fry. Then add this to the rest of the sauce mixture and toss.

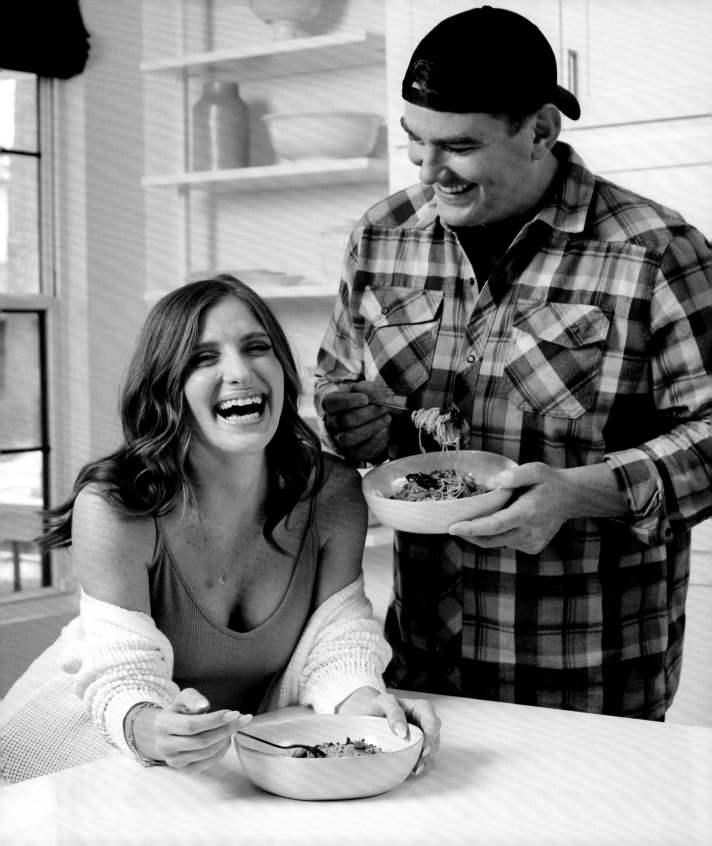

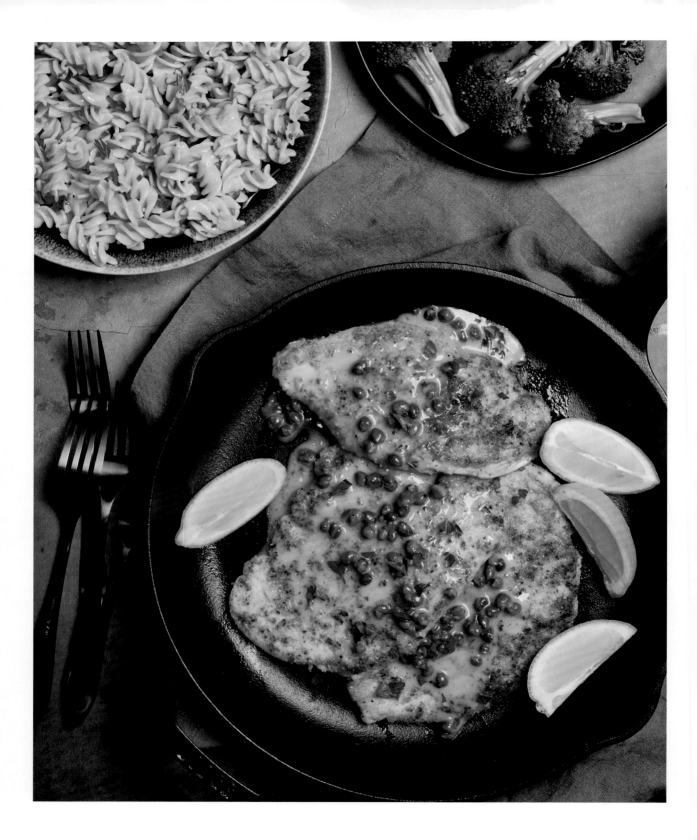

CHICKEN PICCATA

SERVES: 4
PREP TIME: 20 minutes
COOK TIME: 20 minutes

2 boneless, skinless chicken breasts

½ cup almond flour

4 tsp arrowroot starch

Zest and juice of 2 lemons, divided (We love lemon! Halve this if desired.)

Salt and pepper, to taste

2–4 tbsp extra-virgin olive oil (plus more as needed, especially if using a cast-iron pan)

½ cup white wine or chicken broth

¼ cup dairy-free butter

½–1 cup chicken broth

2 tbsp capers, drained, divided

3 tbsp chopped flat-leaf parsley, divided

Gluten-free brown rice pasta (such as Jovial); cauliflower rice; or chopped, steamed broccoli tossed in olive oil and fresh lemon juice (our favorite), for serving

RACHAEL: There's probably no other dish that reminds me more of my grandma than her chicken piccata. A mother of six, she was always in the kitchen. A baker, cook, and outstanding host, she was and still is a force to be reckoned with. Chicken piccata was by no means her signature dish, but it was the first recipe she tried to teach me, and I still remember following her around the kitchen learning to dredge the chicken in flour and how to brown it. Served simply with a butter, lemon juice, and caper sauce, she told me this was an elegant dish I could make for my husband one day. Little did grandma know that I would be marrying the cook and he would be the one making the dish for me.

1 Slice the chicken breasts in half widthwise into 4 cutlets, place cutlets between 2 layers of plastic wrap or parchment paper, and lightly pound each piece very thin (about ½ inch/1.25cm).

2 In a medium bowl, combine the almond flour, arrowroot starch, half of the lemon zest, and salt and pepper to taste. Dredge the chicken in the flour mixture.

3 In a large pan, heat the olive oil over medium-high heat. Add the chicken in batches, and cook for 4 to 5 minutes per side, or just until cooked through. Remove from the pan and set aside.

4 To the same pan, add the wine and deglaze. Add the butter to the pan and melt. Stir to combine. Gradually stir in the chicken broth.

5 Add all of the lemon juice, remaining zest, and 1 tablespoon capers. Reduce the heat to medium-low, and simmer for 3 minutes, stirring occasionally.

6 Return the chicken to the pan. Simmer for 2 to 3 minutes. Stir in 1 teaspoon parsley. Serve with your desired side. Top with the remaining capers and parsley, and enjoy.

NOTE

We prefer this cooked in cast iron for an extra-crisp coating and extra juicy chicken.

MACARONI SALAD

SERVES: 6–8
PREP TIME: 20 minutes, plus 1 hour or overnight to chill
COOK TIME: 10 minutes

8 oz (225g) gluten-free elbow pasta (such as Jovial or Barilla)

1 tsp extra-virgin olive oil

4–6 sweet gherkins, diced (reserve juice for the dressing)

½ red bell pepper, diced

1–2 celery ribs, thinly sliced

⅓ cup diced red onion

2 hard-boiled eggs, roughly chopped

½ cup shredded carrots

Dressing:

1 cup mayonnaise

2 tbsp sweet pickle juice

1½ tbsp red wine vinegar

1 tbsp honey

4 tsp Dijon mustard

¼ tsp salt

¼ tsp pepper

½ tsp garlic powder

⅛ tsp smoked paprika

1 tsp celery seed

TOM: Going gluten-free and dairy-free, sometimes there are dishes we come across that we're bummed we can't have. And then the moment hits when I say to myself, "*Oh wait, that wouldn't be hard to re-create.*" This macaroni salad was one of those epiphanies.

1 Cook the elbow pasta according to the package instructions (less 2 minutes; see note). Drain and rinse immediately with cold water. Add pasta to a large bowl and drizzle with the olive oil. Gently stir so the noodles don't stick together as they sit.

2 To the large bowl, add the pickles, bell pepper, celery, onion, eggs, and carrots. Stir until well combined.

3 Prepare the dressing. In a medium bowl, whisk together all ingredients until well combined.

4 Pour the dressing over the pasta, and gently toss until well combined. For the best flavor, cover the bowl and chill for at least 1 hour or overnight. Stir once more before serving, and enjoy.

NOTE

Check the pasta before the box instructions say to—the noodles can crumble or turn soggy quickly, so we always test 2 minutes before the recommended cook time and then every 30 seconds thereafter.

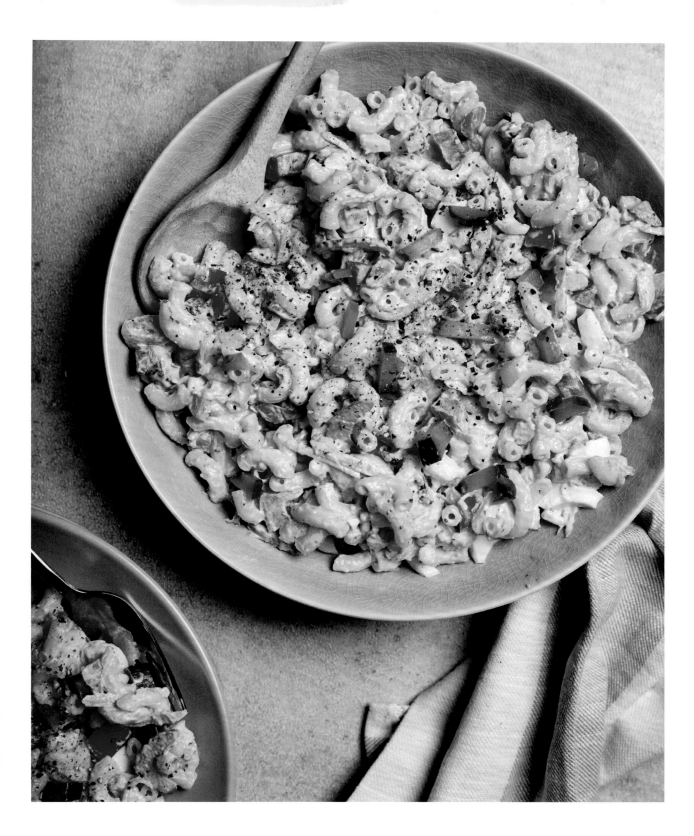

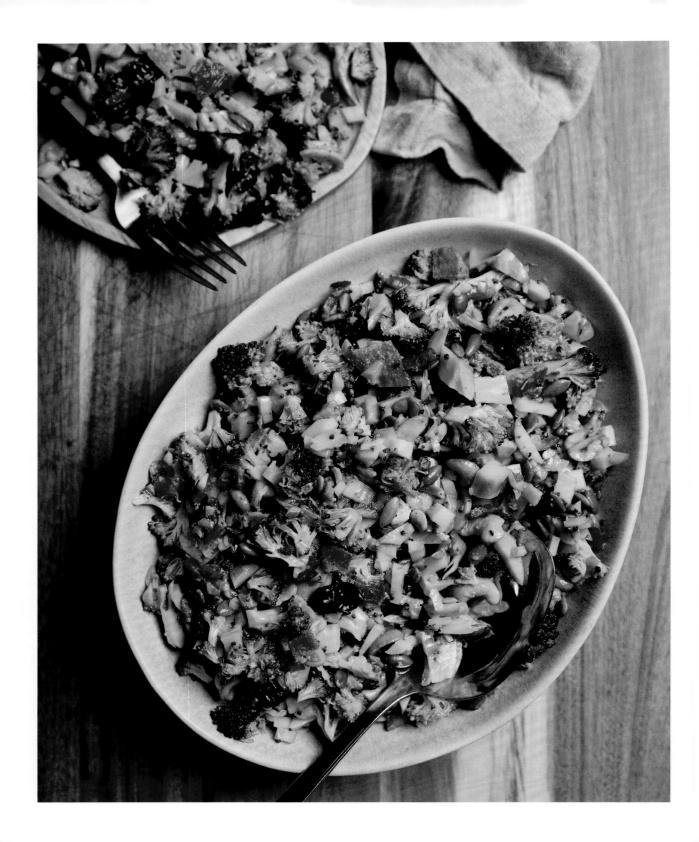

BROCCOLI SALAD

SERVES: 6–8
PREP TIME: 30 minutes
COOK TIME: 4 minutes

½ cup raw seeds, such as pumpkin seeds or flaxseeds

½ cup crushed raw nuts, such as cashews or almonds

1 lb (450g) broccoli florets, chopped

½ cup finely chopped red onion

⅓ cup dried cranberries or dried cherries

3 strips bacon, cooked and crumbled

Honey Mustard Dressing:

⅓ cup extra-virgin olive oil

¼ cup apple cider vinegar

3 tbsp Dijon mustard

3 tbsp honey

1 medium clove garlic, minced

1 tsp sea salt

1 tsp freshly cracked black pepper

TOM: We love this dish! It's a simple classic while also being very versatile. You can have it as a side for dinner or a staple for lunch, it travels well, and it's easy to double the recipe and bring to a party or potluck. It's refreshing while also being hearty at the same time. Just be warned that this will become a regularly requested dish if you start to share it. But hey, you might be like me and enjoy that!

1 In a small bowl, combine all of the dressing ingredients. Whisk until the mixture is well blended. Refrigerate for at least 15 minutes.

2 Meanwhile, toast the seeds and nuts. In a medium skillet, spread them in an even layer. Toast over medium heat, stirring frequently (careful, they'll burn!), until the seeds and nuts are turning golden, about 2 to 4 minutes. (Err on pulling them off early rather than late.) The light toasting draws the oils out (flavor) and decreases moisture (extra crunch). Pour the toasted seeds and nuts into a large serving bowl, reserving some for garnish.

3 Add the broccoli, onion, cranberries, and bacon to the serving bowl.

4 Pour the dressing over the salad, and fold until all of the ingredients are lightly coated in dressing. Chill for 20 minutes to allow the flavors to marry, garnish with reserved nuts, and enjoy.

NOTE

If you want a stellar presentation, serve the salad the same day you make it while the colors are vibrant. It's still great to enjoy all week, but the colors will dull the day after you make it.

CARROT NOODLES
WITH SPICY CASHEW SAUCE

SERVES: 3–5
PREP TIME: 15 minutes
COOK TIME: 20 minutes

2 tbsp toasted sesame oil

2 tsp minced garlic

1 tsp minced fresh ginger or
2 tsp ground ginger

½ tsp crushed red pepper

1 medium red bell pepper, cut into
thin strips

2 cups trimmed sugar snap peas
(optional), sliced on the diagonal

1–2 cups vegetable broth

⅓ cup cashew butter (almond or
peanut butter work, too)

1½ tbsp coconut aminos

Juice of 1 lime

3–5 carrots, spiralized or cut into
medium ribbons

2 cups small broccoli florets

2 green onions, sliced, divided

2 tsp chopped, dry-roasted, salted
cashews

TOM: Full disclosure: we hate zoodles. We just don't like them one bit. They get soggy and don't absorb flavor, in our opinion. If you love them, then go for it! Whether you love or hate them, this is just completely different, so give it a go. The carrots really absorb the liquid very well, but they still have a nice bite to them. I can cook this quickly in 20 minutes or let it sit and thicken, and warm it up later without ruining the integrity of the meal. If you don't have a spiralizer, I use a little handheld one that is under $10, and you are able to knock out three to five carrots quickly.

1 In a large skillet, heat the sesame oil over medium-high heat. Add the garlic, ginger, and crushed red pepper. Cook, stirring constantly, for 30 seconds.

2 Add the bell pepper and snap peas, and cook for 3 minutes or until the peppers are tender, stirring occasionally.

3 Increase the heat to high. In a small bowl, stir together the broth, cashew butter, coconut aminos, and lime juice. Add the mixture to the pan. Bring to a boil and reduce liquid by half.

4 Reduce the heat to medium, and add the carrot noodles, broccoli, and half of the green onions to the skillet. Toss the ingredients, cover, and cook for 3 to 5 minutes or until the carrots are tender-crisp. (Cook for an additional 1 to 2 minutes for more tender noodles.)

5 Uncover and toss to coat the carrot noodles with the mixture. Cook, uncovered, for 2 minutes or until the sauce thickens slightly.

6 Use tongs to plate and ladle on extra sauce if desired. Top with the remaining green onion and the chopped cashews. Enjoy immediately.

NOTE
This is an easy recipe to add protein. Throw in some cooked chicken or any cooked ground meat.

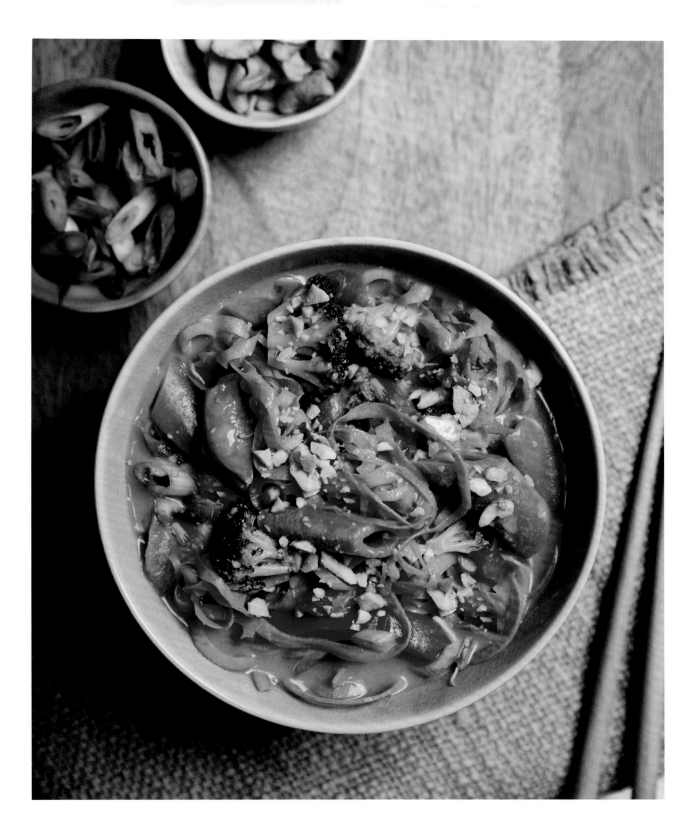

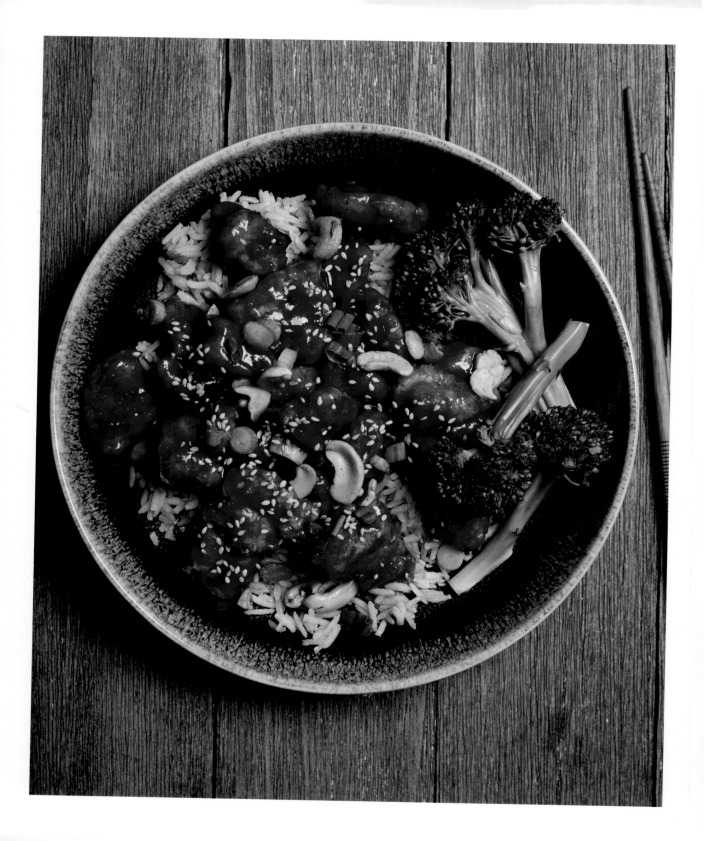

SWEET & STICKY ORANGE CHICKEN

SERVES: 2
PREP TIME: 10 minutes
COOK TIME: 50 minutes if baking
or 25 minutes if frying

¾ cup arrowroot starch

1 tsp salt

1 tsp pepper

2 eggs, whisked (omit if baking)

1 lb (450g) boneless, skinless chicken
  breasts, cut into 1-in (2.5cm) pieces,
  patted dry

½ cup avocado oil, for shallow frying
  (omit if baking)

Brown rice or steamed broccoli,
  for serving

Sliced green onions, sesame seeds,
  and toasted cashews, for garnish

Sauce:

⅔ cup + 1 tsp water, warmed slightly,
  divided

4–6 pitted dates

⅓ cup fresh orange juice

2 tbsp rice vinegar

3 tbsp coconut aminos

½ tsp ground ginger

½ tsp garlic powder

½ tsp crushed red pepper

1 tbsp arrowroot starch

Zest of 1 orange (finely grated)

TOM: My brother Steve came to visit us once and wanted orange chicken for dinner. That sounded easy enough, until I realized typical orange chicken was loaded with ingredients that didn't coincide with Rachael's lifestyle. Nevertheless, we were determined to make a delicious dish that satisfied both Steve's cravings and Rachael's dietary needs . . . and thus this recipe was born.

1 Prepare the sauce. In a food processor, blend ⅔ cup warm water and dates until smooth, about 3 minutes. In a medium saucepan over medium heat, add the orange juice, pitted dates, vinegar, coconut aminos, ginger, garlic, and crushed red pepper. Whisk and heat to a boil, then lower the heat to medium-low. Simmer for 5 minutes.

2 In a small bowl, whisk together the arrowroot starch and remaining water to form a paste. Add to the orange sauce, and whisk well. Raise the heat to medium. Cook for another 2 to 3 minutes or until the mixture thickens. (It should resemble caramel.) Once the sauce is thickened, remove from the heat, stir in the orange zest, and set aside.

3 In a shallow, medium bowl, mix together the arrowroot starch, salt, and pepper. If shallow frying, in a bowl, whisk the eggs and then add the chicken and coat the pieces. Then toss the egg-coated chicken pieces in the arrowroot starch. Place the pieces on a plate.

4 For shallow frying, in a medium skillet, heat the avocado oil over medium-high. Once hot, working in batches, cook the chicken pieces for 7 minutes, flipping once to brown both sides. Place the chicken on a paper towel–lined plate to drain. Repeat in batches for the remaining chicken, adjusting the heat as needed.

5 If baking, preheat the oven to 425°F (220°C). Coat the chicken pieces in the arrowroot mixture. Arrange the chicken pieces on a wire rack over a baking sheet. Bake for 15 to 25 minutes, flip the pieces, and raise the temperature to 450°F (230°C). Cook for 5 to 10 minutes more, or until they reach an internal temperature of 165°F (74°C).

6 Toss the chicken with the sauce. Serve over brown rice or broccoli. Garnish with green onions, sesame seeds, and toasted cashews and enjoy!

CHICKEN
WITH POMEGRANATE & GREEN BEANS

SERVES: 2
PREP TIME: 10 minutes
COOK TIME: 25 minutes

½ lb (225g) boneless, skinless chicken thighs or breasts, cut into bite-size pieces

Salt and pepper, to taste

1 tbsp extra-virgin olive oil, plus more if needed

½ lb (225g) green beans, trimmed, cut into 2-in (5cm) pieces

1 cup pomegranate seeds, divided

2 garlic cloves, minced

2 tbsp or more balsamic vinegar, plus more as desired

2 tbsp toasted sesame oil, plus more as desired

Balsamic glaze (optional), for serving

TOM: This is a classic example of a recipe where we looked at what we should be incorporating during the phase and compared it with what ingredients we had in our house. Rachael was craving both chicken and green beans, and I knew pomegranate would add both a pop of sweetness and a pop of color to this combination. Sometimes making a recipe is that simple. By adding elements like pomegranate and a balsamic glaze, we were able to transform a plain meal into an elevated experience for our palates.

1 In a medium bowl, toss the chicken pieces in salt, pepper, and olive oil. Set aside.

2 Heat a large cast-iron skillet over medium-high heat. Add the green beans. (If not using a cast-iron skillet, toss the green beans gently in a little olive oil.) Cook for 8 to 15 minutes, or until charred and blistered and the desired tenderness, stirring every 2 minutes.

3 Remove the beans from the skillet. Add the chicken to the pan and brown well over medium-high heat, stirring often, for 6 to 7 minutes. Once browned and nearly cooked, add ½ cup pomegranate seeds and the garlic. Cook over medium-high for about 3 minutes until the garlic becomes fragrant and the seeds release some of the juices.
Add the green beans back to the pan, and toss everything together.

4 Add the vinegar and sesame oil. Toss, adding more oil and vinegar as desired. (Watch out for the steam and smoke—get the fan going!)

5 Remove to a serving bowl, and top with the remaining pomegranate seeds. Add a drizzle of balsamic glaze from the pan (if desired), and serve.

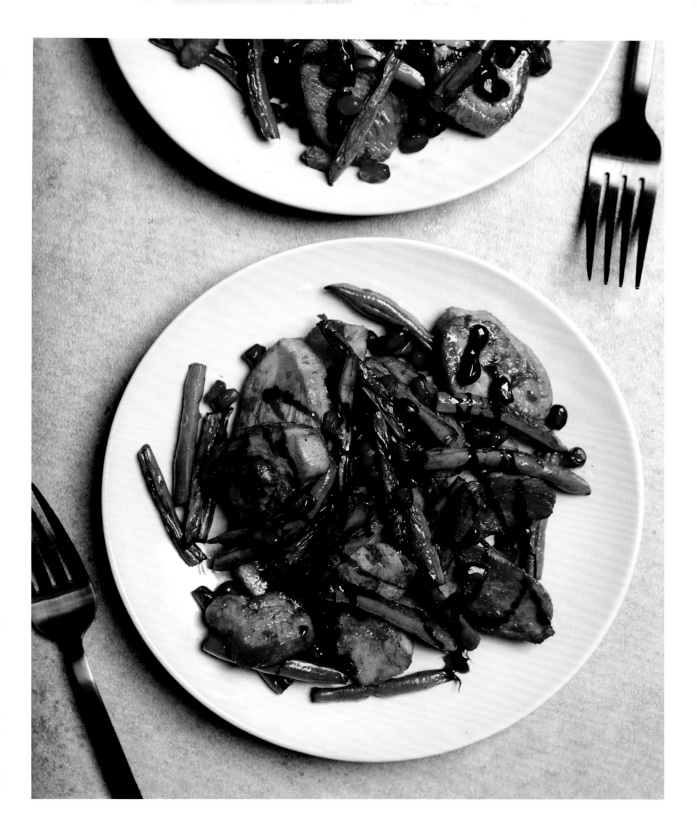

CHAPTER 8

FOODS FOR YOUR OVULATORY PHASE

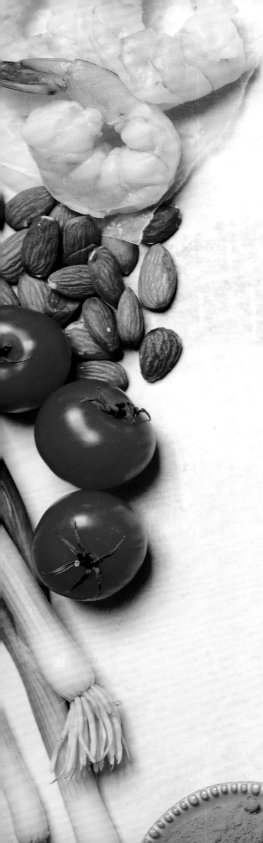

IN THE KITCHEN FOR PHASE 3
OVULATION

During this phase, we want to improve egg quality. Your estrogen reaches its peak levels, triggering the brain to surge with luteinizing hormone (LH), and then ovulation occurs. You may notice an increase in your sex drive. Aphrodisiacs such as dark chocolate, figs, and strawberries are a couple of foods that will help boost the libido. During ovulation, we want to support the liver as it breaks down and removes excess estrogen. To do this, we want to fill up on veggies high in fiber and incorporate foods that boost glutathione levels, the antioxidant required to properly detox every day. This includes asparagus, spinach, and okra. Dandelion is also a superfood during this phase, so this is a good time to try out a new food if you've never had it.

THE PHASE 3 PANTRY

SEEDS

Sesame seeds
Sunflower seeds

NUTS

Almonds
Pecans
Pistachios

GRAINS/BEANS

Corn
Green and red lentils
Quinoa

VEGETABLES

Asparagus
Bell peppers
Brussels sprouts
Chard
Chives
Dandelion greens
Eggplant
Endive
Fennel
Green onions
Okra
Spinach
Tomatoes

FRUITS

Apricot
Cantaloupe
Coconut
Figs
Guava
Raspberries
Strawberries

MEATS/PROTEINS

Lamb

SEAFOOD

Salmon
Shrimp
Tuna

OTHER

Dark chocolate
Ketchup
Turmeric

COOKING METHODS FOR PHASE 3

Our food is digesting great during this phase, and these foods all help create a healthy egg, keep bloating down, keep acne at bay, and flush excess hormones. We are going to eat raw fruits and vegetables, such as hearty salads. Cooking techniques such as steaming, poaching, blending, and juicing promote healthy digestion and detoxification.

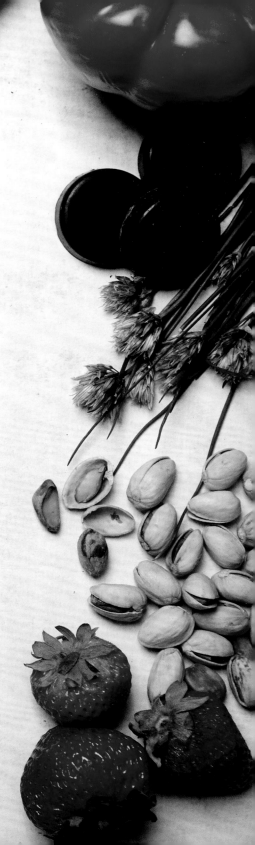

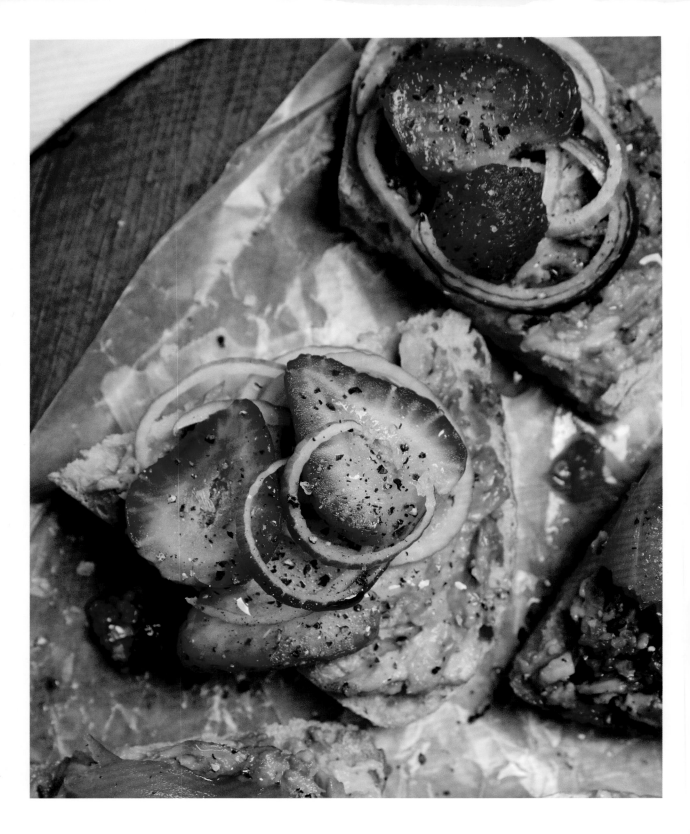

AVOCADO TOAST
WITH STRAWBERRY & ONION

SERVES: 1
PREP TIME: 5 minutes
COOK TIME: 2 minutes

2 slices gluten-free bread

½ avocado

¼ red onion, or to taste, thinly sliced

2–3 strawberries, thinly sliced

1 tsp extra-virgin olive oil

Freshly cracked black pepper, to taste

Salt, to taste

RACHAEL: We spent 4 years living in downtown Chicago, in the neighborhood of Bucktown. Less than a 5-minute walk in every direction were restaurants, bars, and little neighborhood cafés, one in particular being Red June Cafe. Tucked off the main street, located on the first floor of a duplex, Red June is a quaint local neighborhood spot where everyone knows the owner, Kim, by name. It has a walkup window on the side of the building where they serve dog treats to all the four-legged friends. It holds the charm and character I love about Chicago. On their menu is an avocado toast topped with red onions and strawberries that tastes like a version of a spinach and strawberry salad. Immediately hooked on the flavors, we've been recreating the meal at home ever since.

1 Toast the bread. Place the avocado on the toasted bread. Smash with a fork and spread over the toast.

2 Arrange the red onions over the avocado. Top with the strawberry slices.

3 Drizzle the olive oil over the top, and sprinkle with the pepper and salt. Enjoy.

AVOCADO TOAST
WITH SMOKED SALMON

SERVES: 1
PREP TIME: 5 minutes
COOK TIME: 2 minutes

2 slices gluten-free bread

½ avocado

2 pieces smoked salmon (we prefer hot-smoked or cured lox)

2 tbsp chili crisp, such as Fly by Jing or homemade

Freshly cracked black pepper, to taste

Salt, to taste

RACHAEL: Tom's first time to Europe was the winter of 2018 when we explored Sweden together for 10 days. We spent an evening in an igloo underneath the Northern Lights, an afternoon dog sledding in the untouched wilderness of the Arctic circle, and days wandering the city centers taking part in *fika,* a typical Swedish tradition where you allow yourself a moment in time, a break from the day to pause and enjoy a hot drink and a snack with friends. Tom and I loved to fika. While most people snacked on baked goods or sweet treats, Tom's rendition of fika was indulging in pickled and smoked fish, a craving that we brought back home with us to the States. This smoked salmon and chili oil toast was inspired by that trip and even after one bite, this dish has a way of transporting us back to those European winter days.

1 Toast the bread. Place the avocado on the toasted bread. Smash with a fork and spread over the toast.

2 Arrange the smoked salmon on top of the avocado.

3 Drizzle with the chili oil, and finish with pepper and salt. Enjoy.

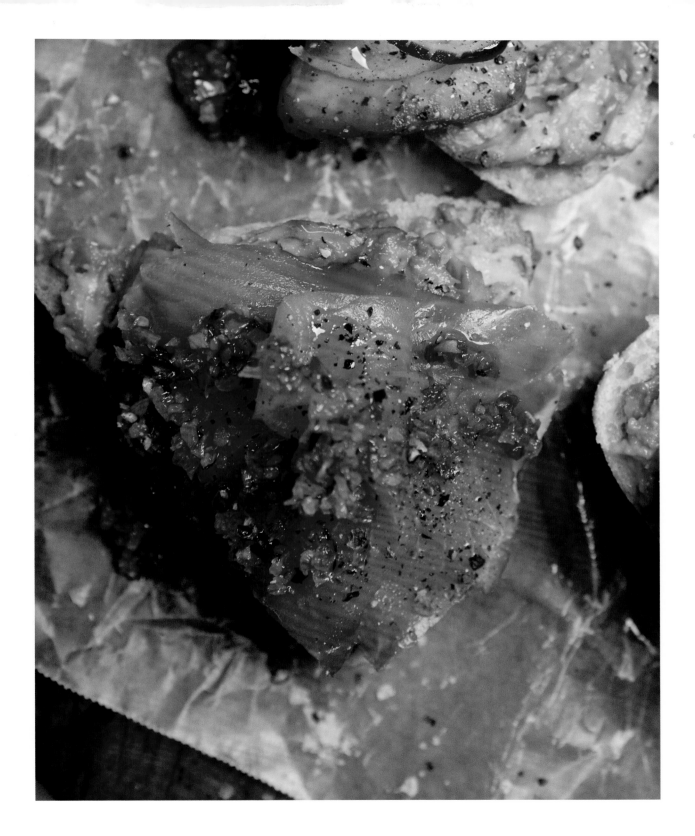

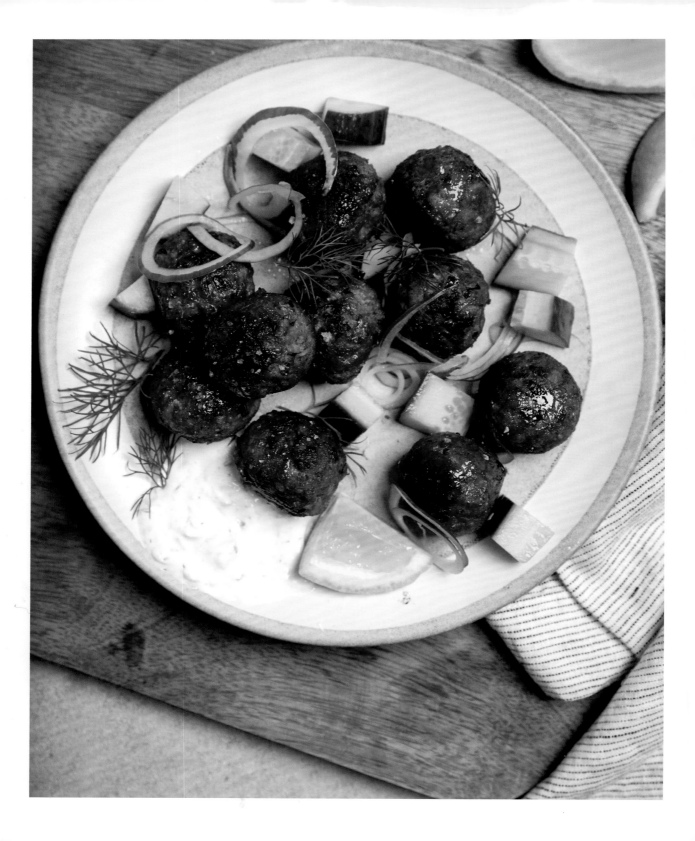

LAMB MEATBALLS
WITH VEGAN TZATZIKI

SERVES: 3–4
PREP TIME: 15 minutes, plus
15 minutes or overnight to chill
COOK TIME: 40 minutes

Tzatziki:

1½ cups grated cucumber (no need
   to peel or seed)

1 cup plain dairy-free yogurt

2 tbsp chopped fresh dill or
   1½ tbsp ground dill

1 tbsp lemon juice

1 garlic clove, minced

1 tsp salt

Meatballs:

1 lb (450g) ground lamb

1 white onion, grated or finely diced

½ cup gluten-free breadcrumbs

1 large egg

⅓ cup finely chopped cilantro

1 tsp ground cumin

1 tsp smoked paprika

Zest of ½ lemon

½ tsp ground cinnamon

Dash of cayenne

Salt and pepper, to taste

1 tbsp extra-virgin olive oil

RACHAEL: When we decided to honeymoon in New Zealand, I missed the part during my research where the country's population was overrun by lamb. Lamb shank, lamb lollipops, meat pies, roasted leg of lamb—there was a lamb recipe for every occasion. These lamb meatballs, although cooked Mediterranean style, come from the adventures we shared in New Zealand on our honeymoon, and now we get to share a part of that experience with you.

1 Prepare the tzatziki. Place the grated cucumber in a strainer to drain for about 10 minutes. Use your hands to squeeze out extra moisture.

2 In a small bowl, stir together the yogurt, dill, lemon juice, garlic, and salt. Stir in the cucumber. Taste and adjust seasonings. Cover and refrigerate for 15 minutes or overnight.

3 For the meatballs, in a large bowl, mix everything except the olive oil. Form into meatballs. We prefer to make tablespoon-size meatballs (or a smaller-size cookie scoop). The smaller size allows them to cook quicker. This yields 20 to 25 small meatballs or about 12 medium-to-large meatballs.

4 In a large pan, heat the oil over medium-high heat. (It should be hot enough that the meatballs sizzle when they hit the pan.) Cook in batches, turning until browned on all sides and cooked through, about 8 to 10 minutes. Transfer to a plate and serve with the tzatziki.

SERVING SUGGESTIONS
Enjoy as a salad with red onion and cucumber, as an appetizer with sauce for dipping, in a gluten-free gyro, or over rice.

OVEN OPTION
Preheat the oven to 400°F (200°C). Arrange the meatballs on a baking sheet. Cook for 20 minutes, turning once halfway through.

PECAN-CRUSTED SALMON

SERVES: 4
PREP TIME: 5 minutes, plus
30 minutes to 2 hours to chill
COOK TIME: 10 minutes

½ cup chopped raw pecans

1 tsp smoked paprika

1 tsp chipotle powder

½ tsp onion powder

1½ tbsp pure maple syrup

1 tbsp apple cider vinegar

1 tsp coconut aminos

4 skin-on salmon fillets
  (about 6 oz/170g each)

Salt and pepper, to taste

1 tbsp dairy-free butter

Sautéed sliced brussels sprouts,
  leeks, or spinach, tossed in a
  drizzle of maple syrup, for serving

TOM: Rachael had sent me a photo from St. Thomas sitting on the beach, under a palm tree in her bikini, snacking on none other than my pecan-crusted salmon. Talk about my idea of a centerfold. This was one of her many work trips as a flight attendant where I would help her meal prep. I remember she was on call that month, meaning she didn't know where the airline would send her, so we loaded her up with several days' worth of food. It wasn't every day she landed a Caribbean layover, so I assumed she would have taken advantage of the location and gone out for fresh seafood. But she didn't. She chose to eat my salmon instead . . . at least that's the story the picture tells.

1 In a small bowl, stir together the pecans, paprika, chipotle powder, onion powder, maple syrup, apple cider vinegar, and coconut aminos.

2 Pat the fillets dry with paper towels, and sprinkle salt and pepper on each. Spoon and press the pecan mixture evenly onto each fillet. Refrigerate, covered, for at least 30 minutes and up to 2 hours.

3 Remove the salmon from the refrigerator. Preheat the oven to 425°F (220°C).

4 In a large cast-iron or oven-safe skillet, melt the butter over medium-high heat. When the pan is hot, add the salmon skin-side down. Sear, undisturbed, for 2 minutes.

5 Transfer the pan to the oven and cook for 6 to 9 minutes, depending on the thickness, until the internal temperature reaches 125°F (52°C). Remove from the oven and let it rest until the temperature comes up to 135°F (57°C), and enjoy.

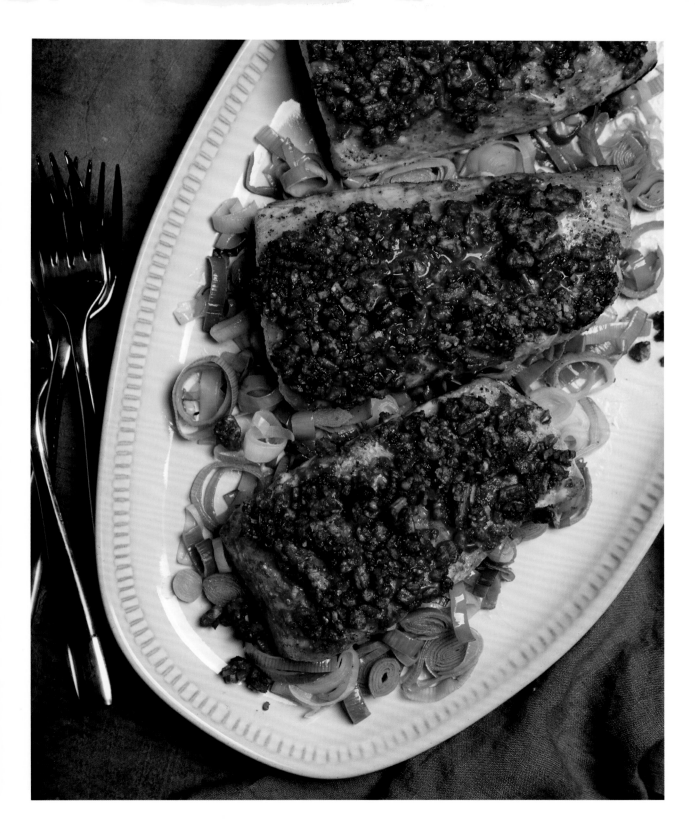

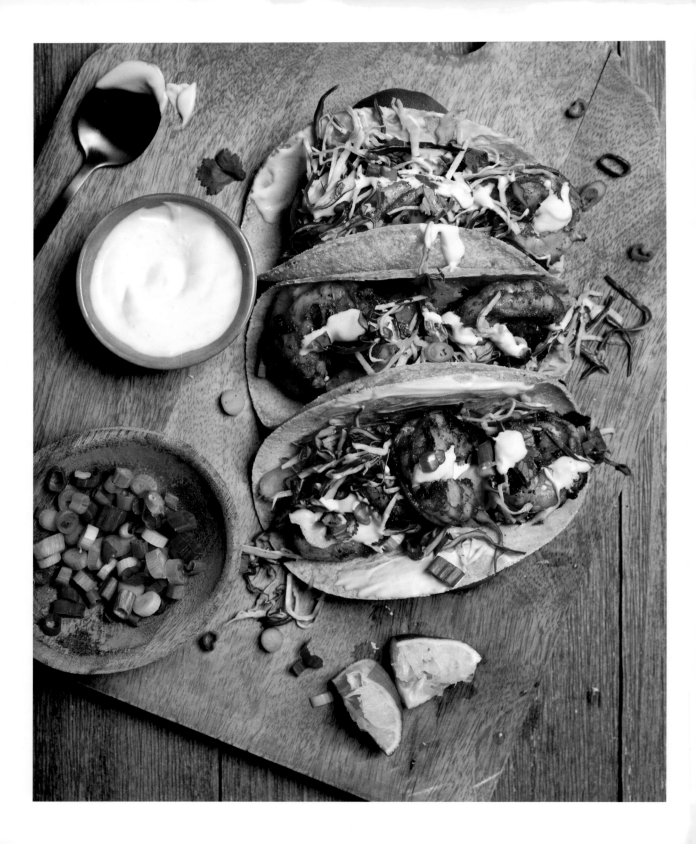

BLACKENED SHRIMP TACOS
WITH CABBAGE SLAW

SERVES: 3–5
PREP TIME: 20 minutes
COOK TIME: 8 minutes

8 corn tortillas
Sliced green onions, for garnish

Slaw:
2 cups shredded red or
  green cabbage
Juice of ½ lime
¼ cup chopped cilantro
¼ tsp salt, or to taste
¼ tsp pepper, or to taste

Spicy Mayo:
½ cup mayonnaise
Juice of ½–1 lime
2 tbsp sriracha
¼ tsp salt

Shrimp:
1 lb (450g) peeled and deveined
  fresh shrimp
2 tsp chili powder
2 tsp smoked paprika
1 tsp ground cumin
1 tsp garlic powder
1 tsp onion powder
½ tsp freshly ground black pepper
½ tsp salt
¼ tsp cayenne
1 tbsp extra-virgin olive oil

TOM: A particular ingredient I have learned to fall in love with is cabbage. Not only is it inexpensive, but it's also packed with vitamins and nutrients, promotes digestion, and improves heart health among a list of other benefits. I feel like it should make the superfoods list! These blackened shrimp tacos are topped with a cabbage slaw and spicy mayo that will leave your tastebuds looking for additional ways to utilize these ingredients in other recipes.

1 In a medium bowl, combine all of the ingredients for the slaw. Cover and refrigerate. (This can be made a day or two ahead.)

2 In a small bowl, whisk together all of the ingredients for the spicy mayo. Cover and refrigerate until ready to use. (This can also be made a day or two ahead.)

3 In a medium bowl, toss the shrimp with the dried spices.

4 In a large cast-iron skillet, heat the olive oil over medium-high heat, swirling the skillet to coat the bottom. Add the shrimp and sear for 2 to 4 minutes per side, or until slightly blackened.

5 Assemble the tacos. Warm the tortillas. Spread spicy mayo over the tortillas, and add 3 to 4 shrimp to each. Top each with about ¼ cup slaw and another 1 tablespoon spicy mayo. Garnish with green onions. Fold the tacos and enjoy.

CITRUS BRUSSELS SALAD

SERVES: 4–6
PREP TIME: 30 minutes
COOK TIME: 15 minutes

TOM: I grew up only knowing brussels sprouts to be cooked one way: boiled in a steamed bag and then topped with what felt like a gallon of melted cheese. Over the last decade, brussels sprouts have really made a name for themselves in the restaurant industry. Now regularly seen on menus, they are being served anywhere from raw and crunchy to roasted and crispy. To honor this new generation of how brussels sprouts are prepared, this dish features a medley of savory, bright, and piquant flavors that accommodate the raw, shredded sprouts. And because cruciferous vegetables, like brussels sprouts, are known to lower insulin resistance, your hormones will be happy with you.

6–8 slices bacon

1½ lb (680g) brussels sprouts, shredded (either use a food processor, or roll up your sleeves and slice thinly)

½ cup slivered or sliced almonds, toasted

1 cup dried cranberries or cherries

1 small red onion, thinly sliced

Citrus Vinaigrette:

Zest and juice of 1 small orange

Juice of 1 lemon

2 tbsp finely minced shallot

1 garlic clove, minced

1 tbsp honey mustard

½ cup extra-virgin olive oil

2 tsp finely chopped fresh thyme leaves or 1 tsp dried thyme leaves

Salt and pepper, to taste

1 In a large bowl, whisk together all of the ingredients for the citrus vinaigrette. Cover and refrigerate.

2 In a large pan over medium heat, cook the bacon until crispy. Allow to cool, and crumble. Stir the bacon into the vinaigrette and let sit for at least 10 minutes before adding the other ingredients to the bowl.

3 Add the brussels sprouts, almonds, cranberries, and red onion to the bowl of vinaigrette. Toss to coat well. Serve and enjoy.

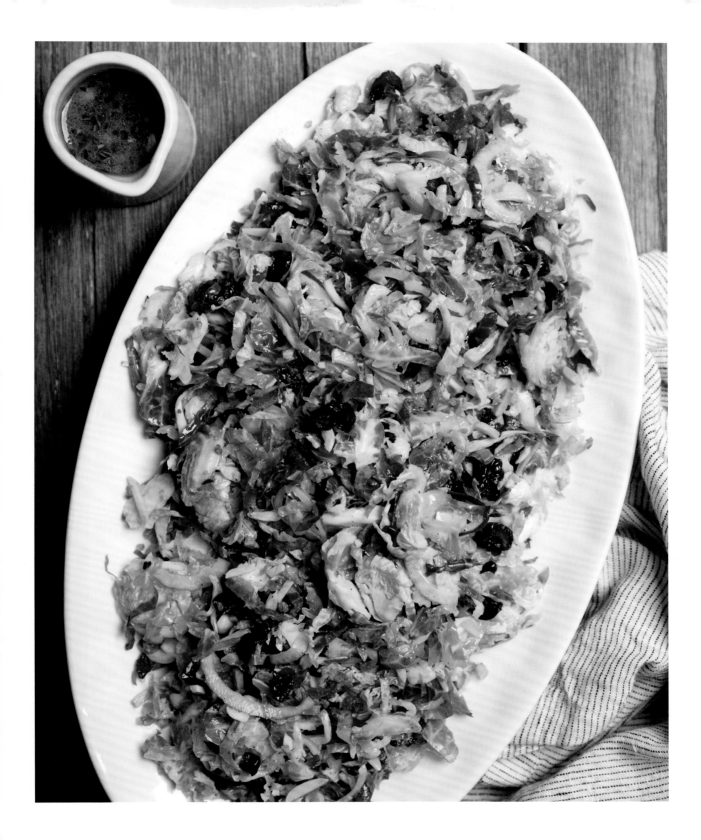

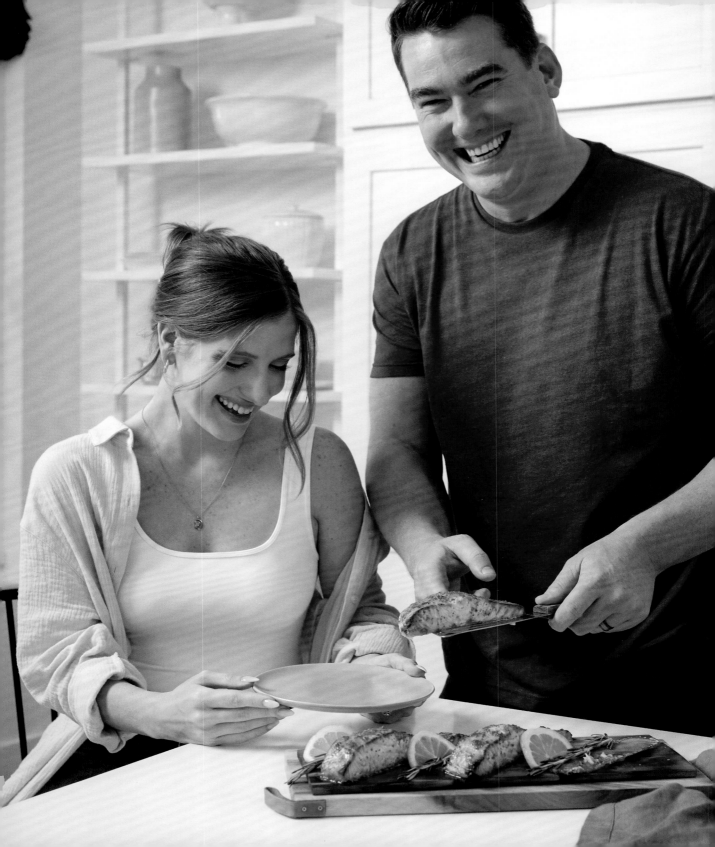

CEDAR PLANK SALMON

SERVES: 2
PREP TIME: 30 minutes to 1 hour, plus soaking the plank
COOK TIME: 15 minutes

1 cedar grilling plank

2 tbsp stone-ground or grainy mustard

1 tbsp honey mustard

2 tbsp honey

1 tbsp finely chopped rosemary

Zest and juice of ½ lemon

1 tsp salt

Freshly cracked black pepper, to taste

¾ cup arrowroot starch

1 (2 lb/900g) skin-on Alaskan salmon fillet (about 1½ in/3.75cm thick), cut to fit the cedar plank

OVEN OPTION

Do steps 1 through 4. Preheat the oven to 350°F (180°C). Place a rack on a baking sheet (feel free to line with foil). Place the plank on the rack. Bake for 20 to 25 minutes or until the salmon flakes easily or reaches 140°F (60°C).

RACHAEL: It was my 23rd birthday, and I had worked an afternoon flight from LA to Chicago while Tom was at home prepping a surprise birthday dinner for me. Instead of asking what food I was in the mood for, he asked me what I wanted to drink. This man was working in reverse to create a whole meal around what I wanted to drink, and that was sexy. I was in the mood for a glass of white wine, so we picked up some Oyster Bay sauvignon blanc from New Zealand, which turned out to be the same winery we would later visit on our honeymoon. And then he made grilled cedar plank salmon with—*oh my gosh*—the most delicious rosemary honey glaze. This salmon is arguably one of my favorite dishes he makes and a staple to have paired with a bottle of Oyster Bay.

1 Submerge the cedar plank in water and soak for 30 minutes to 1 hour.

2 Preheat the grill to medium-high heat (450–550°F/230–290°C). Every grill is different, but for ours, we use indirect heat by turning the middle burner off and leaving the others on. If using a charcoal grill, use indirect heat, as well.

3 In a small bowl, stir together the stone-ground mustard, honey mustard, honey, rosemary, lemon zest and juice, salt, and pepper.

4 Place the salmon on the plank, skin-side down. Spread the mustard mixture all over the salmon and let stand at room temperature for 15 minutes.

5 Place the plank on the grill (over the burner that's not turned on, if applicable), and close the lid. Try to resist opening the lid! Grill until the salmon is just cooked through and the edges are browned, about 13 to 15 minutes. You should smell the cedar charring. The plank may catch fire; gently mist the fire with water or blow it out. If you don't smell the plank, you may want to turn the burner below it on low. Once the salmon flakes easily or reaches 140°F (60°C), remove it. Let the salmon stand on the plank for about 5 minutes before serving.

CHAPTER 9

FOODS FOR YOUR LUTEAL PHASE

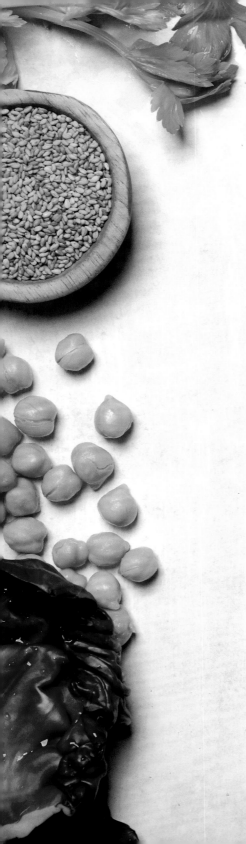

IN THE KITCHEN FOR PHASE 4
LUTEAL

During the luteal phase, it's important to aid in progesterone production and prioritize blood-sugar balance. At the end of this phase, your progesterone production stops, which brings on your period. Supporting progesterone production up until then will help to relieve PMS symptoms. Foods containing vitamins and minerals such as magnesium, zinc, B_6, B_9, and E have been shown to increase progesterone. To aid in blood-sugar balance, we want to make sure we don't skip any meals, stay hydrated, and choose balanced meals that contain complex carbohydrates, fiber, protein, and fat.

THE PHASE 4 PANTRY

SEEDS

Sesame seeds
Sunflower seeds

NUTS

Hickory nuts
Pine nuts
Walnuts

GRAINS/BEANS

Brown rice
Chickpeas
Navy beans

VEGETABLES

Cabbage
Cauliflower
Celery
Collard greens
Cucumber
Daikon
Garlic
Ginger
Leek
Mustard greens
Onions
Parsnip
Pumpkin
Radish
Shallots
Squash
Sweet potatoes
Watercress

FRUITS

Apples
Bananas
Dates
Peaches
Pears
Raisins

MEATS/PROTEINS

Beef
Turkey

SEAFOOD

Cod
Flounder
Halibut

OTHER

Mint
Peppermint
Spirulina

COOKING METHODS FOR PHASE 4

When preparing these foods, think about warm foods in order to help your digestive tract absorb the nutrients. Roasting and baking are going to be the best methods, and enjoying a warm beverage after a meal is a great way to aid digestion.

SWEET POTATO HASH

SERVES: 4
PREP TIME: 15 minutes
COOK TIME: 40 minutes

3 strips bacon, cut into ½-in (1.25cm) pieces

4 oz (115g) ground breakfast sausage

1 medium sweet potato, cut into ½-in (1.25cm) cubes

1 tsp smoked paprika

1 tsp salt

1 tsp pepper

1 medium onion, roughly chopped

1 medium bell pepper (any color), roughly chopped

4 large eggs

Avocado or olive oil, as needed

Optional toppings: thinly sliced green onions, hot sauce, sauerkraut, roasted red peppers, and avocados

RACHAEL: If you're lucky enough to stay at Sullivan's Bed and Breakfast (that's our guest bedroom), eating will be the most memorable experience of your trip. As a master host, Tom has the smell of breakfast circulating the room before you even wake up. It sometimes feels like a sprint to get out of bed just to see what he's put together. A traditional breakfast of choice is his sweet potato hash.

I find this dish to be the converter of the non–sweet potato believers. My dad, for example, doesn't care for sweet potatoes, but he really enjoys this recipe to the point that he goes back for seconds. It's such a simple dish, but the presentation has you feeling like you've been served by a private chef in the Hamptons, and the flavors match.

1 Heat a medium cast-iron skillet over medium heat. Add the bacon and sausage. Cook until the sausage is cooked three-fourths through, breaking it up as it cooks. Remove meats to a plate. Preheat the oven to 400°F (200°C).

2 Raise the heat on the stove to medium-high. Add the sweet potatoes to the skillet. Stir to coat the potatoes in the bacon oil, and then stir in the smoked paprika, salt, and pepper. We like our potatoes crispy on the outside and soft in the middle, so we allow them to sit undisturbed until a crust forms, about 7 to 10 minutes, depending on your skillet. If you like the potatoes softer, just cover the skillet after adding the spices, and cook over medium heat for 7 to 10 minutes.

3 Once the sweet potatoes are nearly cooked to desired tenderness, add the onion and pepper. Cook for an additional 2 to 4 minutes, stirring occasionally, until the onions and peppers are soft and fragrant. Add the meat back in, and stir to combine. Create 4 wells where you will crack each egg. Carefully crack an egg into each space.

4 Put the skillet into the preheated oven. Bake the eggs to your preference, about 5 minutes for a runny yolk, 10 minutes for a medium yolk, and 15 minutes for a hard yolk. Serve with the desired toppings.

NOTE

We like to add leftover meats to this recipe--brisket, pulled pork, or chicken are all great. Add your leftover meats in step 3, when you add the bacon and sausage back to the skillet.

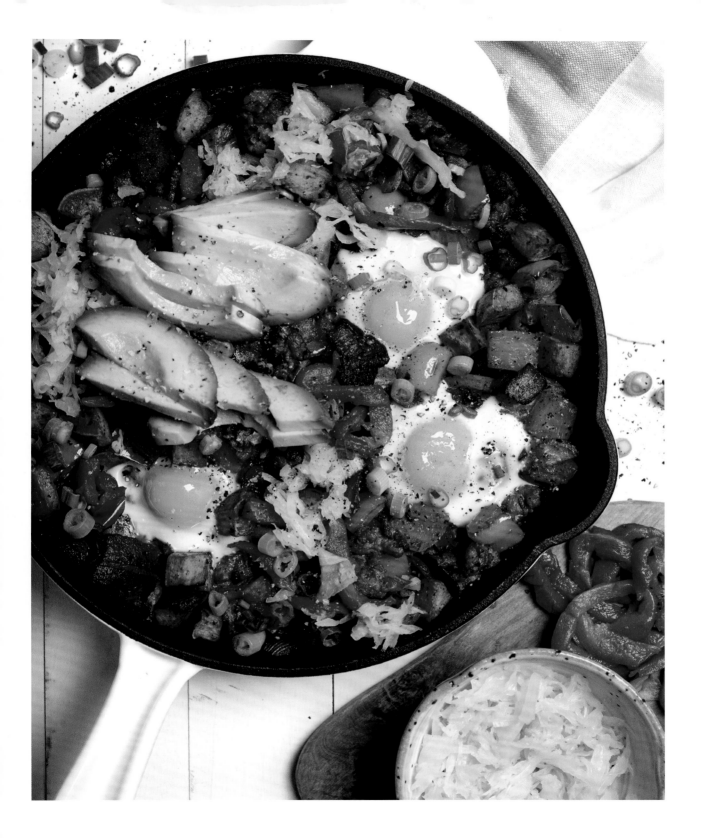

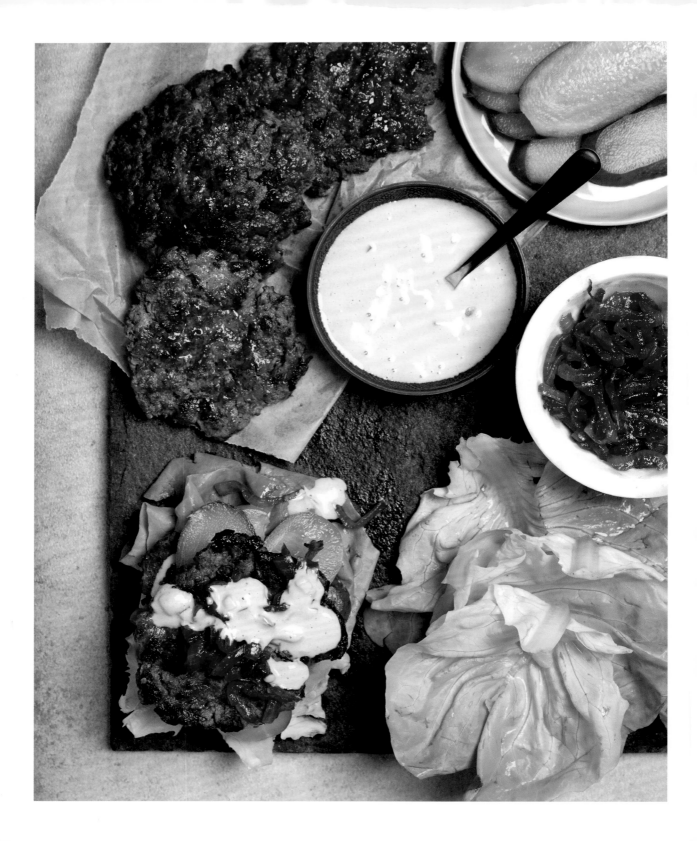

SMASH BURGERS ANIMAL STYLE

SERVES: 4
PREP TIME: 15 minutes
COOK TIME: 50 minutes

1 tsp seasoned salt

1 lb (450g) ground beef

3 tsp avocado oil or extra-virgin olive oil

¼ cup yellow mustard

8 leaves of iceberg or Bibb lettuce (for "buns")

Sandwich pickles, to serve

Animal Sauce:

½ cup mayonnaise

3 tbsp ketchup

2 sandwich pickles, diced

1 tbsp coconut aminos

½ tsp apple cider vinegar

Caramelized Onions:

1 tbsp extra-virgin olive oil

1 tbsp dairy-free butter

1 white onion, cut into half rings

1 tsp seasoned salt

RACHAEL: I don't know how I went 20 years without ordering a burger at a restaurant. Maybe it's because my parents cooked 80 percent of our meals or the fact that when we did go out as a family, we exclusively went out for Italian food. That spell was finally broken when Tom took me to the University of Illinois, his old stomping grounds, and introduced me to Seven Saints, an American-style tavern for creative burgers. I lost my burger virginity that weekend and I'm here to say, if you've never grilled a burger on your own, we're honored to be your first.

1 Make the sauce. In a small bowl, whisk together all of the ingredients. Cover and refrigerate until ready to use.

2 Caramelize the onions. In a nonstick pan, heat the oil and butter over medium heat. Once the butter is melted, add the onion and salt. Reduce the heat to medium-low, stirring occasionally, for about 45 minutes, or until the onions are golden and caramelized. Stir in 1 to 2 tablespoons water to rehydrate as needed. Let cool.

3 While the onions are caramelizing, form the patties. In a large bowl, use your hands to mix together the seasoned salt and ground beef. Form into 8 (2-oz/57g) balls.

4 Heat a griddle or cast-iron skillet over medium-high heat. Once hot, add the avocado oil to your griddle. When the oil is very hot, work in batches and add the burger patties. Immediately smash the patties with a spatula to get them thin. Spread ½ tablespoon mustard on the top, raw-side of each patty. Cook the patties, undisturbed, until they're very well-browned and a bit crusty on the bottom, about 2 to 3 minutes. Flip the patties so the mustard side is down, and cook for 1 minute more.

5 Assemble your burgers. For each burger, spread a tablespoon of animal sauce onto the inside of one lettuce "bun." Then layer a burger patty, animal sauce, caramelized onions, pickles, and another burger patty. Top with more onions and animal sauce. Top with another leaf of lettuce bun. Grab napkins and enjoy!

JIBARITO

SERVES: 4–5 sandwiches
PREP TIME: 15 minutes, plus 1 hour or overnight to marinate and chill
COOK TIME: 25 minutes

1 lb (450g) iron, flank, or hanger steak

2 (7 oz/200g) cans chipotle peppers in adobo, divided

2 cloves garlic, minced, divided

2 tsp honey, divided

1 cup mayonnaise

2 green plantains

1 cup extra-virgin olive oil or avocado oil

Himalayan salt, to taste

¼ red onion, sliced into rounds

1 heirloom tomato, sliced

Arugula, to top

RACHAEL: The jibarito is a Puerto Rican–inspired dish that was first introduced in Chicago exactly one left turn and 3 miles up the road from where we lived. This dish spread like wildfire across the local Puerto Rican restaurants, one of which was La Cocina Boricua, where Tom and I tried the sandwich for the first time. This sandwich soon became a craving I couldn't shake, and when I get a craving, Tom gets inspired. We know you'll absolutely love our version of the jibarito and if you don't, we promise a money-back guarantee on this book. For legal reasons, that's a joke, but we know you won't be disappointed.

1 Place the steak and 1 can chipotle peppers in adobo in a resealable bag, squishing to break up the peppers. Add 1 clove minced garlic and 1 teaspoon honey. Fill the empty adobo can with water, and pour into the bag. Seal the bag and marinate steak in the refrigerator for at least 1 hour or overnight.

2 In a small bowl, stir together the mayonnaise, adobo sauce from the remaining can of chipotle peppers, and remaining garlic and honey. Cover and refrigerate. Save the remaining peppers, if desired.

3 Bring a medium pot of water to a boil. Peel the plantains. Cut each one into 4 to 5 chunks about 1-inch (2.5cm) thick. Place the pieces in the boiling water and cook for 3 to 6 minutes, until they turn deep yellow. Remove with a slotted spoon. Place the segments between two pieces of parchment paper. Flatten the slices, one at a time, pressing with a pot or bowl.

4 Preheat the grill to medium-high. Meanwhile, in a large skillet over medium-high heat, heat the oil until it reaches 350°F (180°C). Line a plate with paper towels. Working in batches, use a slotted spatula to lift the flattened plantain pieces and place in the preheated oil. Cook for 1 to 3 minutes, flip, and cook for another 1 to 3 minutes until the edges start to brown. Remove to the plate. Season with salt.

5 Grill the steak to the desired temperature. Allow to rest for at least 10 minutes. Slice thinly against the grain.

6 To assemble each jibarito, spread the sauce on both sides of the plantain "bun." Layer the steak, red onion, tomato slices, and arugula into the sandwich. Enjoy!

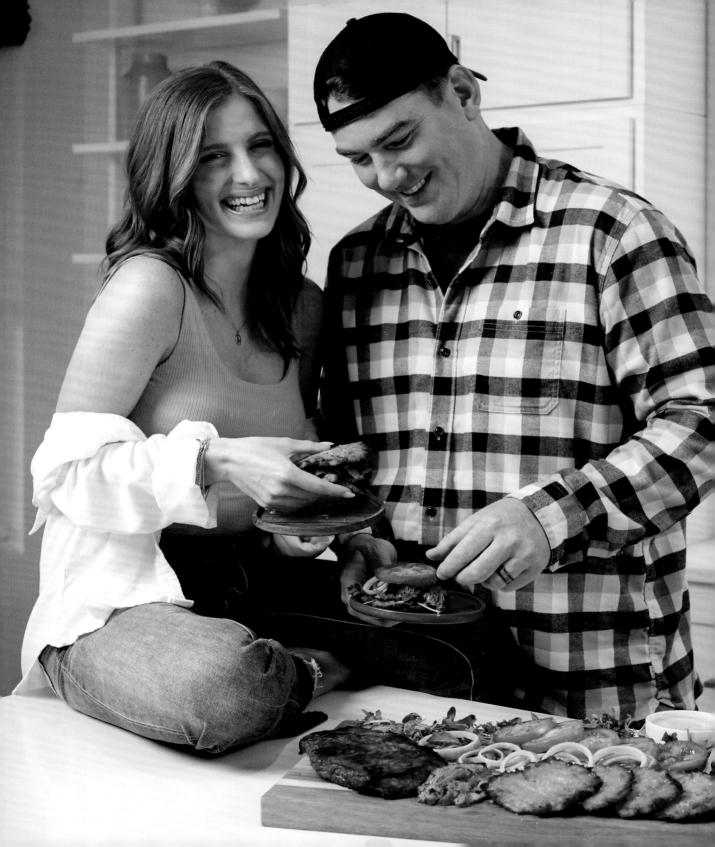

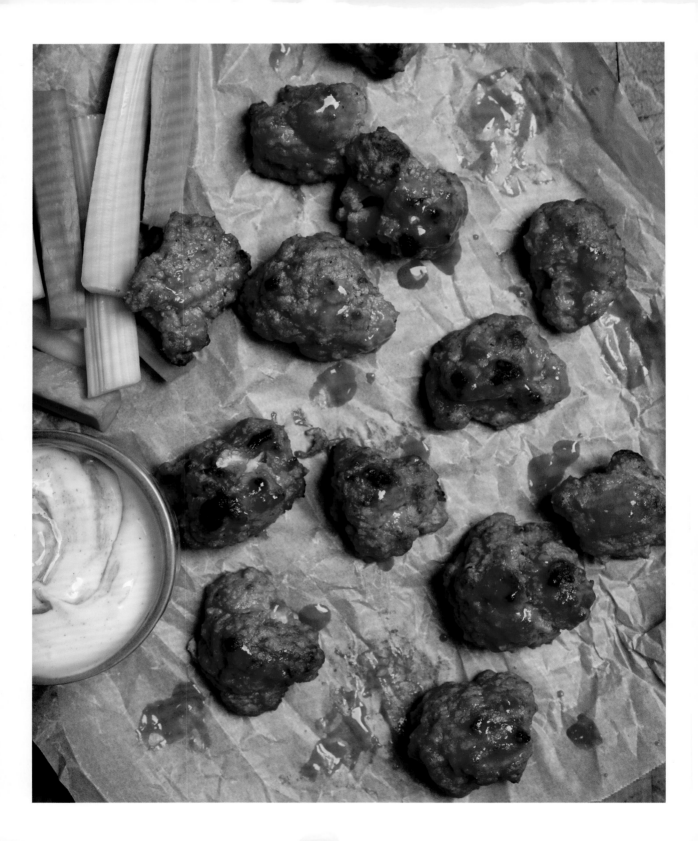

BUFFALO CAULIFLOWER "WINGS"

SERVES: 2
PREP TIME: 10 minutes
COOK TIME: 30 minutes

3 tbsp arrowroot starch

2 tsp garlic powder

2 tsp onion powder, divided

1 tsp salt

1 tsp freshly ground black pepper

2 large eggs

1 tbsp water

1 head of cauliflower, chopped into bite-size pieces

¼ cup dairy-free butter

2 cloves garlic, minced

2 cups hot sauce

Dairy-free ranch (such as Hidden Valley Plant Powered) and celery, for serving

RACHAEL: We have a group of friends very near and dear to our hearts who we refer to as the Super Bowl Crew. One of those crew members, Colleen, is vegetarian. A few years ago during our annual Super Bowl party, Tom wanted to make sure Colleen felt included with all the tailgate favorites, so he prepared for her these buffalo cauliflower wings. We know the pain of showing up to a party and there's nothing that fits your dietary needs. We also know how grateful we are when people are conscious of that. I can promise you these wings will be beloved by all, and the only reason I can say that so matter-of-factly is because my Uncle Duane, Uncle Mark, and Uncle Mike devoured most of the cauliflower wings that Super Bowl Sunday before Colleen could even go back for seconds.

1 Preheat the oven to 450°F (230°C). Line a baking sheet with parchment paper, and place a wire rack on top. Spray the rack with nonstick cooking spray. (If you don't have a wire rack, turn the pieces once halfway through cooking.)

2 In a medium bowl, stir together the arrowroot starch, garlic powder, 1 teaspoon onion powder, salt, and pepper. In another bowl, whisk together the eggs and water. Toss the cauliflower pieces in the egg mixture, then roll them in the dry mixture.

3 Arrange the seasoned cauliflower on the wire rack. Bake for 20 to 25 minutes, or until the desired doneness. (We like them crispy with a bit of browning on the edges.)

4 Meanwhile, prepare your sauce. In a small saucepan, melt the butter with the minced garlic over medium heat. Add the hot sauce and remaining onion powder. Whisk well, and simmer for 5 minutes. Then reduce the heat to low until the cauliflower pieces are done.

5 Remove the cauliflower from the oven and preheat the broiler. Whisk the hot sauce to make sure it's well combined. Toss the cauliflower "wings" until coated. (I prefer to use tongs and dunk them each into the sauce.) Arrange on the prepared rack and broil for 2 to 4 minutes. Serve immediately.

CHICKPEA SALAD

SERVES: 6–8
PREP TIME: 30 minutes, plus
30 minutes to chill
COOK TIME: 2 minutes

3 tbsp extra-virgin olive oil

2 tbsp red wine vinegar

2 tbsp honey

2 garlic cloves, minced

2 tsp fresh or dried basil, plus leaves
for garnish

Zest and juice of 1 lime

1 tsp salt

1 tsp freshly cracked black pepper

3 cups cooked chickpeas or
2 (15 oz/425g) cans chickpeas,
drained and rinsed

1 red bell pepper, diced

2 celery ribs, diced

½ yellow squash, diced

½ large red onion, thinly sliced

1 cup red cabbage, chopped
(about ¼ head of cabbage)

½ cucumber, diced

TOM: This salad is perfect for the luteal phase. As you get closer to menstruation and you may not be in the mood to cook, this easy dish is the nutrition your body craves, and it's easy on your digestive system. This recipe is loaded with seven of the ingredients from your luteal phase list. Chickpea salad is a great side for a barbecue, hearty enough for a meal, or as Rach would tell you from experience as a flight attendant, "the perfect 4-hour weather-delay snack." We dare you not to fall in love with this one.

1 To a medium saucepan, add the olive oil, red wine vinegar, honey, garlic, basil, lime zest and juice, salt, and pepper. Whisk over medium-low heat until combined. Then remove pan from the heat and allow to cool.

2 To a large serving bowl, add the chickpeas, bell pepper, celery, squash, red onion, cabbage, and cucumber. Toss to combine.

3 Pour the cooled dressing over the salad. Toss to coat. Cover and refrigerate for at least 30 minutes or until ready to serve. Eat within 5 days.

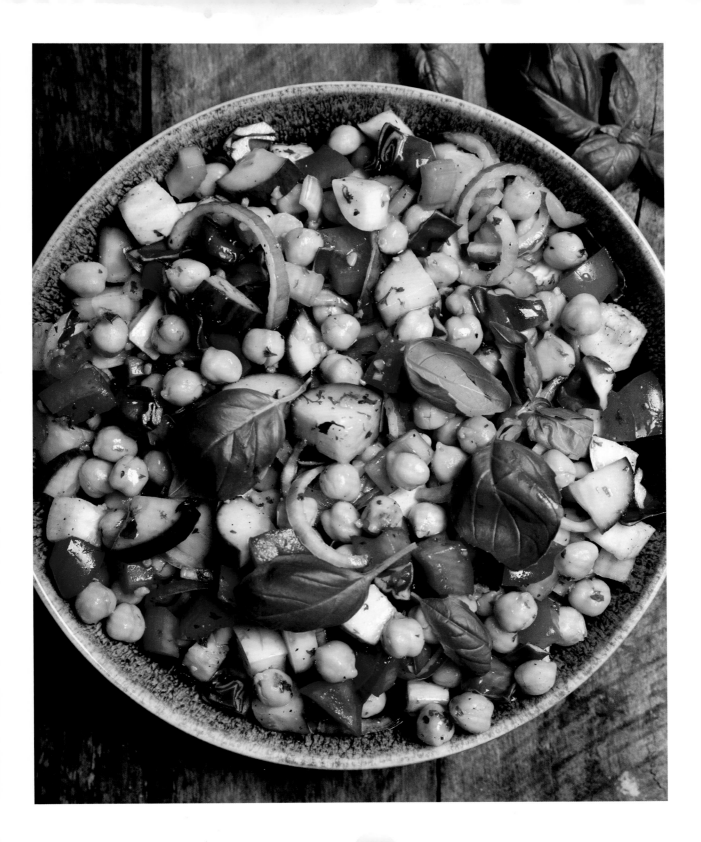

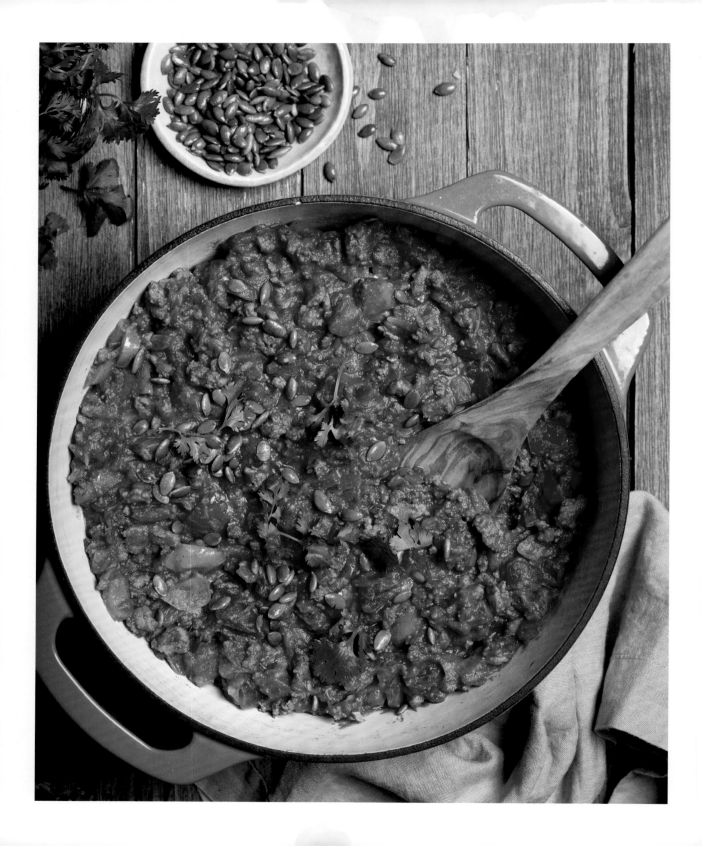

PUMPKIN TURKEY CHILI

SERVES: 6
PREP TIME: 15 minutes
COOK TIME: 35 minutes

1 tbsp extra-virgin olive oil

1 medium white onion, diced

1 medium red bell pepper, diced

1 medium yellow bell pepper, diced

1 lb (450g) ground turkey

½ tbsp garlic powder

½–1 tbsp chili powder (to taste; we prefer more)

½ tsp ground cinnamon

Salt and pepper, to taste

1 (15 oz/425g) can diced tomatoes

1 (15 oz/425g) can pumpkin purée

Toasted pumpkin seeds, dairy-free sour cream, and fresh cilantro, for serving

RACHAEL: After the *Rachael Ray Show* got word of Tom's secret Instagram account, which was created as a space to organize all these recipes, Rachael had us on the show for an interview and to share our story. We left that episode speechless as they gifted us with a year of organic groceries to keep inspiring Tom in the kitchen. Tom's inspiration expanded to not only me and my needs, but soon the needs of the community. A month after we were on the show, our local college cafeterias were shut down as a result of COVID-19. That's when we started making homemade meals for a certain college student, better known on the internet as College Kid Kevin. What started as feeding one college student turned into feeding thousands more when we claimed we had adopted him, and by that I meant we gave him free food. We opened our home and Rachael Ray's wallet to the local college community and used the free groceries she gave us to make biweekly to-go meals out of our kitchen. Each meal had a theme, and when fall was approaching, we decided to do a chili cook-off against ourselves. With over eight different chili recipes, Tom included a chili to correspond with my cycle, and that was when this pumpkin turkey chili recipe was born.

1 In a deep skillet, Dutch oven, or large pot, heat the oil over medium heat. Cook the onion and bell peppers, stirring often, until the onion is translucent, about 5 minutes

2 Turn the heat to medium-high, and add the ground turkey. Cook until browned, breaking it up with a wooden spoon as it cooks, about 7 minutes.

3 Add the garlic powder, chili powder, cinnamon, salt, and pepper. Stir continuously for 1 minute.

4 Stir in the diced tomatoes with their juice and the pumpkin purée. Bring the mixture to a simmer for 20 minutes. If it gets too thick, stir in 1 to 2 cups water or vegetable stock, a ¼ cup at a time, until the desired consistency is achieved. Serve with toasted pumpkin seeds, dairy-free sour cream, and cilantro.

INDEX

RESOURCES

FOODS FOR THE
MENSTRUAL PHASE

SEEDS

Flaxseeds
Pumpkin seeds

NUTS

Brazil nuts
Chestnuts

GRAINS/BEANS

Chickpeas
Green lentils
Kidney beans
Wheat germ
Wild rice

VEGETABLES

Arugula
Beets
Chard
Kale
Kelp
Mushrooms
Spinach
Sweet potatoes

FRUITS

Blackberries
Blueberries
Cranberries
Grapes
Pineapple
Prunes
Watermelon

MEAT/PROTEINS

Duck
Lean pork (tenderloin, boneless top loin, or sirloin roast)
Tofu

SEAFOOD

Clams
Crab
Lobster
Mussels
Octopus
Oysters
Salmon
Scallops

OTHER

Bone broth
Dark chocolate
Light teas (nettle, raspberry leaf, chamomile, and ginger)
Miso
Probiotic yogurts (dairy-free)
Salt
Turmeric

FOODS FOR THE
FOLLICULAR PHASE

SEEDS

Flaxseeds
Pumpkin seeds

NUTS

Brazil nuts
Cashews

GRAINS/BEANS

Brown rice
Lima beans
Oats
Quinoa

VEGETABLES

Artichoke
Broccoli
Bibb, Boston, buttercrunch, butterhead, or four seasons
  lettuce
Carrots
Edamame
Parsley
Peas
Rhubarb
Zucchini

FRUITS

Avocado
Grapefruit
Lemon
Lime
Orange
Plums
Pomegranate

MEATS/PROTEIN

Chicken
Eggs

SEAFOOD

Trout

OTHER

Apple cider vinegar
Kimchi
Nut butter
Olives
Pickles
Sauerkraut

FOODS FOR THE
OVULATORY PHASE

SEEDS

Sesame seeds
Sunflower seeds

NUTS

Almonds
Pecans
Pistachios

GRAINS/BEANS

Corn
Green and red lentils
Quinoa

VEGETABLES

Asparagus
Bell peppers
Brussels sprouts
Chard
Chives
Dandelion greens
Eggplant
Endive
Fennel
Green onions
Okra
Spinach
Tomatoes

FRUITS

Apricot
Cantaloupe
Coconut
Figs
Guava
Raspberries
Strawberries

MEATS/PROTEINS

Lamb

SEAFOOD

Salmon
Shrimp
Tuna

OTHER

Dark chocolate
Ketchup
Turmeric

FOODS FOR THE
LUTEAL PHASE

SEEDS

Sesame seeds
Sunflower seeds

NUTS

Hickory nuts
Pine nuts
Walnuts

GRAINS/BEANS

Brown rice
Chickpeas
Navy beans

VEGETABLES

Cabbage
Cauliflower
Celery
Collard greens
Cucumber
Daikon
Garlic
Ginger
Leek
Mustard greens
Onions
Parsnip
Pumpkin
Radish
Shallots
Squash

VEGETABLES, CONTINUED

Sweet potatoes
Watercress

FRUITS

Apples
Bananas
Dates
Peaches
Pears
Raisins

MEATS/PROTEINS

Beef
Turkey

SEAFOOD

Cod
Flounder
Halibut

OTHER

Mint
Peppermint
Spirulina

28-DAY MEAL GUIDE

This is our example of what 28 days of meals could look like, not a hard and fast meal plan. If you're not sure what phase you're in or where to start, see page 79. Remember that every single food on these lists, no matter the phase, is beneficial to your health, so you can, and absolutely should, overlap them.

When cooking, we often make extra and use the leftovers the following day to create new dishes or to eat for lunch. You'll also see ingredients on the phase list that were used for dinner make their way into egg dishes for the next breakfast or incorporated into lunch. In the span of a month, we're definitely ordering to-go food and enjoying meals out as well.

In the guide below, salads, yogurt bowls, and smoothies are left as general terms so you can incorporate several items from the food list that you enjoy. For our personal favorite yogurt bowls and sheet pan meals, see pages 103 to 105.

MENSTRUATION: 5 DAYS

Reminders: get plenty of rest; keep your iron and zinc intake up

Cooking methods: try to avoid whole, raw fruits and veggies; juicing and smoothies are great options; warm, well-cooked foods will be desired

Add-ons: hot leaf teas

Snacks: dark chocolate, fruit

Day 1
Breakfast: smoothie

Lunch: soup with a protein (meat or chickpeas)

Dinner: baked crab legs (such as page 117)

Day 2
Breakfast: yogurt bowl (such as on page 103)

Lunch: spinach and mushroom soup

Dinner: sheet pan meal (such as on pages 104 and 105) with sweet potato fries

Day 3
Breakfast: smoked salmon and a bowl of fruit

Lunch: miso soup (such as on page 110)

Dinner: crab cakes (such as on page 121)

Day 4
Breakfast: scrambled eggs with mushrooms and spinach

Lunch: roasted beets over arugula and baked salmon

Dinner: balsamic pork (such as on page 118) with sweet potato fries

Day 5
Breakfast: smoothie

Lunch: beet salad (such as on page 114)

Dinner: pork stew (such as on page 113)

FOLLICULAR PHASE: 10 DAYS

Cooking methods: steaming and sautéing
Reminders: stay hydrated; enjoy a wide variety of foods
Add-ons: water with apple cider vinegar and honey
Snacks: hard-boiled eggs, pickles, pumpkin seeds

Day 6
Breakfast: nut butter toast and fruit
Lunch: chicken soup
Dinner: carrot noodles (such as on page 134)

Day 7
Breakfast: eggs and fruit
Lunch: broccoli salad (such as on page 133)
Dinner: quinoa with avocado and chicken

Day 8
Breakfast: yogurt bowl (such as on page 103)
Lunch: macaroni salad (such as on page 130)
Dinner: chicken piccata (such as on page 129)

Day 9
Breakfast: veggie omelet
Lunch: leftovers
Dinner: sautéed trout with peas

Day 10
Breakfast: yogurt bowl (such as on page 103)
Lunch: leftovers (soup, macaroni, or broccoli) with trout or chicken
Dinner: stir-fry with chicken

Day 11
Breakfast: overnight oats
Lunch: grilled chicken with steamed broccoli and balsamic vinegar
Dinner: pasta (such as on page 126)

Day 12
Breakfast: nut butter toast and fruit
Lunch: brown rice with sautéed veggies
Dinner: sheet pan chicken (such as on page 105) with brown rice

Day 13
Breakfast: scrambled eggs with avocado
Lunch: leafy green salad with grilled chicken
Dinner: bibimbap (kimchi over brown rice)

Day 14
Breakfast: avocado toast (such as on pages 144 and 146)
Lunch: leftovers
Dinner: chicken with green beans (such as on page 138)

Day 15
Breakfast: smoothie
Lunch: leafy green salad with hard-boiled eggs and veggies
Dinner: sweet and sticky orange chicken (such as on page 137) over brown rice

OVULATION: 3 DAYS

Reminders: detox/eliminate used hormones; with estrogen at an all-time high, eat foods that support your liver
Cooking methods: steaming, blending, poaching, and juicing
Add-ons: turmeric shot, clean juices
Snacks: almonds, pistachios

Day 16 (overlap with follicular)
Breakfast: smoothie
Lunch: spinach salad with grilled salmon
Dinner: pecan-crusted salmon (such as on page 150) with steamed brussels sprouts

Day 17
Breakfast: poached egg over spinach and steamed asparagus
Lunch: blackened shrimp salad
Dinner: lamb meatballs with tzatziki (such as on page 149), lentils, and cucumber salad

Day 18
Breakfast: smoothie
Lunch: citrus brussels salad (such as on page 154)
Dinner: cedar plank salmon (such as on page 157)

LUTEAL PHASE: 11 DAYS

Reminders: prioritize warm foods in order to help the digestive tract

Cooking methods: roasting and baking

Add-ons: warm beverages, such as ginger tea, after meals

Snacks: dates with nut butter, beef sticks

Day 19 (overlap ovulation)
Breakfast: smoothie

Lunch: leafy green salad

Dinner: lamb meatballs with brown rice and chickpeas

Day 20
Breakfast: banana with nut butter

Lunch: ground beef burger bowl with coleslaw

Dinner: pumpkin turkey chili

Day 21
Breakfast: yogurt bowl (such as on page 103)

Lunch: chickpea salad (such as on page 170)

Dinner: sheet pan meal (such as on pages 104 and 105)

Day 22
Breakfast: sweet potato hash (such as on page 162)

Lunch: leftovers

Dinner: smash burgers (such as on page 165) with coleslaw

Day 23
Breakfast: leftovers

Lunch: ground turkey with coleslaw

Dinner: baked halibut with sweet potato fries

Day 24
Breakfast: smoothie

Lunch: ground turkey stir-fry

Dinner: baked cod with mustard greens

Day 25
Breakfast: yogurt bowl (such as on page 103)

Lunch: daikon radish and cucumber salad

Dinner: turkey meatloaf with sweet potato fries

Day 26
Breakfast: apple with nut butter and protein bar

Lunch: leftovers

Dinner: buffalo cauliflower "wings" (such as on page 169)

Day 27
Breakfast: banana with nut butter

Lunch: leftovers

Dinner: jibaritos (such as on page 166)

Day 28
Breakfast: eggs with fruit

Lunch: Korean ground beef and rice bowl

Dinner: oven-roasted beef with roasted vegetables

ACKNOWLEDGMENTS

TOGETHER: Our dog and first "child" Odin, thank you for sacrificing so many walks in order for us to meet deadlines, as well as for late nights up past your bedtime, keeping you awake as we type away.

Mike and Judy Gallagher, a huge thank you for being a constant balance when the stress became too much. Oh, and for always being on call to help us find the bottom of a bottle of wine.

Katie Krasowski: Thank you for being our fashion eye and helping Rachael pick out outfits while 4 months pregnant. Even more importantly, for making sure she knew she looked amazing for the photo shoot for this book.

For all the reviewing, input, and overall support—a big thank you to Traci and George. Being a sounding board during this process made it possible to get this work complete.

Lauren Tully, for always checking in and being a constant anchor of support. Being a call or text away to get a quick brainstorm meant the world.

The whole DK team who worked on the book production, we literally couldn't have pulled this through without you. Thank you for making this possible and pulling it all together. Brandon Buechley, for keeping us organized and for that smile you bring on every call. Becky Batchelor, for your creativity and flexibility.

A special thanks to Alexandra Andrzejewski, for the knowledge and commitment you bring to the table regarding PCOS, as well as your passion to bring more resources and light to this topic.

Everyone at Indy for the photo shoot! You made it a seamless and enjoyable experience. We can't thank you enough. The entire crew made a whole day of pictures, outfit changes, and what would seem to be chaos go not just smoothly but truly enjoyable. And to Kelley Schuyler and your amazing photography skills!

Thank you, Chef Ashley Brooks and stylist Lovoni Walker for sharing your incredible skills and insight with us. You are true masters at your crafts.

A special shout out to food stylist Chung Chow for not only making the food look amazing, but also for lending your necklace to Rachael for the photo. Oh, and having such a great taste in fashion!

A huge thank you for lending your wealth of knowledge to us and not having an ego while doing it, we want to thank Dr. Bryson Whalen. Giving us the amount of time you did was amazing, and sharing insight of what it feels like being on your side of the PCOS discussion will be beneficial to so many! Thank you, again.

Our Southside crew! Thank you, Denise Ferguson and Shannon Schickel, coming through on hair and make-up for the photo shoot and making Rachael look like the queen that she is. You nailed every single detail! Your energy and attention to detail helped make the day go smoothly and kept our energy where it needed to be. You both rock!

Thank you, Michael and Hannah Jones, as well as the whole J1S team for being by our side every step of the way. A special shout out to Bridget O'Leary for going above and beyond to help us get this book over the finish line. You wore many hats through this project. No question it wouldn't have come together the way we envisioned without you.

TOM: Lenore Sullivan, my mom, thank you for your support and for trying your best to ask the questions that Dad and I would have talked back and forth about for hours.

And to my beautiful and gifted wife, Rachael. While "we" wrote this together, there is no doubt that it's your creative touch that will make people smile, and your openness to share your life—genuinely and transparently—that will bring hope, courage, closure, and confidence to so many who will read this. We started this book when you were 3 months pregnant and handed in our final writing as Sutton just turned 2 months old. Thank you for being the amazing, talented, sexy, funny, and open person you are. And, as always, thank you for making me feel comfortable to just be myself.

RACHAEL: To my husband, Tom. Thank you for all you have done for me, for us, and for our growing family. My love for you has no end.

To my parents, Nanci and Edward Skerrett. During those final weeks of editing, when I just needed my mom or dad to cuddle on the couch with, it was nice having you both by my side.

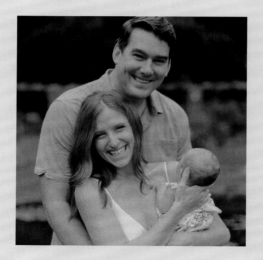

ABOUT THE AUTHORS

Born and raised in Chicago, Illinois, Tom and Rachael Sullivan are the couple behind the social media accounts Meals She Eats and RachSullivan__. They have appeared on *Good Morning America, TODAY Show,* and the *Rachael Ray Show,* and been featured in *USA Today, Parents Magazine, Southern Living, Yahoo, Newsweek,* and more. Tom and Rachael currently reside in North Carolina with their daughter, Sutton, and their perfect pup, Odin. Find them on Instagram @ MealsSheEats and on TikTok @ RachSullivan__.